Cerebral Palsy - Epidemiology, Etiology, Clinical Presentation, Treatments, and Outcomes

Edited by Boulenouar Mesraoua

Published in London, United Kingdom

Cerebral Palsy - Epidemiology, Etiology, Clinical Presentation, Treatments, and Outcomes
http://dx.doi.org/10.5772/intechopen.1001497
Edited by Boulenouar Mesraoua

Contributors
Binjing Dou, Caixia Zhao, Daniela Munoz-Chesta, Juchuan Dong, Lihua Jin, Mónica Troncoso-Schifferli,
N.S. Krishna, Ping He, Ratnadeep Biswas, S.G. Praveen, Ziyad Makoshi

Notice
Statements and opinions expressed in the chapters are these of the individual contributors and not
necessarily those of the editors or publisher. No responsibility is accepted for the accuracy of
information contained in the published chapters. The publisher assumes no responsibility for any
damage or injury to persons or property arising out of the use of any materials, instructions, methods
or ideas contained in the book.

First published in London, United Kingdom, 2025 by IntechOpen
IntechOpen is the global imprint of INTECHOPEN LIMITED, registered in England and Wales,
registration number: 11086078, 167-169 Great Portland Street, London, W1W 5PF, United Kingdom

For EU product safety concerns: IN TECH d.o.o., Prolaz Marije Krucifikse Kozulić 3, 51000 Rijeka,
Croatia, info@intechopen.com or visit our website at intechopen.com.

British Library Cataloguing-in-Publication Data
A catalogue record for this book is available from the British Library

Cerebral Palsy - Epidemiology, Etiology, Clinical Presentation, Treatments, and Outcomes
Edited by Boulenouar Mesraoua
p. cm.
Print ISBN 978-1-83634-563-3
Online ISBN 978-1-83634-562-6
eBook (PDF) ISBN 978-1-83634-564-0

If disposing of this product, please recycle the paper responsibly.

IntechOpen

intechopen.com

Built by scientists, for scientists

Meet the editor

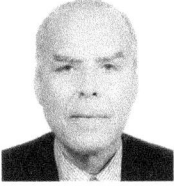

Dr. Boulenouar Mesraoua is a consultant neurologist at Hamad Medical Corporation and an Associate Professor of Neurology at Weill Cornell Medical College, Doha, Qatar. He graduated in Medicine from Algeria, enrolled in a neurology residency program at Liege University in Belgium, had EEG training at the National Hospital for Nervous Diseases in London, UK, and completed a fellowship in epilepsy and EEG monitoring at Zurich University, Department of Clinical Neurophysiology, Switzerland, under the direction of the late Dr. Hans Gregor Wieser. Dr. Mesraoua is currently the Director of the Neurology Fellowship Program and Founder and Director of the Comprehensive Epilepsy Program at Hamad Medical Corporation. He is also the Deputy Director of the residency program at Qatar Medical School. His main interests are epilepsy and clinical neurology.

Contents

Preface

This Edited Volume is a collection of reviewed and relevant research chapters concerning the developments within cerebral palsy. The book features scholarly contributions from various authors and is edited by an expert in the field. Each contribution comes as a separate chapter complete in itself but directly related to the book's topics and objectives.

The book includes the following chapters:

1. Deep Brain Stimulation in Cerebral Palsy

2. Neurosurgical Management of Spasticity

3. Neurodevelopmental, Neurobehavioral, and Psychosocial Aspects of Cerebral Palsy

4. Influence of Robotic Interventions on Gait Improvement in Children with Cerebral Palsy

5. Hand Splinting

The target audience comprises scholars and specialists in the field.

IntechOpen

Chapter 1

Deep Brain Stimulation in Cerebral Palsy

Daniela Munoz-Chesta and Mónica Troncoso-Schifferli

Abstract

Dystonia is a movement disorder defined by involuntary, sustained, or inter-mittent muscle contractions, typically described as repetitive, twisted postures. Dyskinetic cerebral palsy is the most common cause of acquired dystonia in children. Dystonia in patients with cerebral palsy can affect function, pain, comfort, and quality of life. Pharmacological treatment is often unsatisfactory. Deep brain stimulation (DBS), a surgical neuromodulation therapy, has been reported to be an effective treatment for dystonia in patients with cerebral palsy. Multiple clinical variables have been associated with improved outcomes, including diminished disease dura-tion, decreased surgical age, heightened frequency of irregular intraoperative GPi microelectrode firing, and the absence of enduring skeletal abnormalities. These characteristics may operate as positive prognostic indications for the therapeutic effectiveness of DBS. Conversely, large cerebral lesions, the intensity of dystonia, and accompanying spasticity may hinder therapeutic efficacy. At present, there are no defined eligibility requirements for DBS. Evidence indicates that DBS not only facilitates motor enhancements in dystonia in patients with cerebral palsy but also significantly improves quality of life.

Keywords: dystonia, dyskinesia, cerebral palsy, deep brain stimulation, neuromodulation

1. Introduction

The most prevalent non-genetic cause of acquired dystonia is cerebral palsy (CP) [1]. Between 4% and 17% of CP patients experience different dyskinetic move-ment disorders, such as chorea, athetosis, and/or dystonia [2]; these patients are categorized as having dyskinetic cerebral palsy. Dyskinetic cerebral palsy is the most common cause of acquired dystonia in children [1]. Dystonia is defined as "move-ment disorder characterized by sustained or intermittent muscle contractions causing abnormal, often repetitive, movements, postures, or both. Dystonic movements are typically patterned, twisting, and may be tremulous. Dystonia is often initiated or worsened by voluntary action and is associated with overflow muscle activation" [3]. In patients with dystonia secondary to CP, all four extremities are typically involved, with the upper body being most prominently affected. Dystonia in CP patients is associated with pain and musculoskeletal abnormalities, which may have an impact on quality of life and social involvement [4].

The treatment of dyskinetic CP is challenging and pharmacological interventions are frequently ineffective [5]. Deep brain stimulation (DBS), a surgical neuromodulation therapy, has been reported to be an effective treatment for dystonia in patients with CP [6–8].

2. Deep brain stimulation

Deep brain stimulation (DBS) is an effective neuromodulatory therapy that, through the stereotactic implantation of quadripolar electrodes, delivers chronic stimulation to specific intracranial targets. Actually, DBS is widely used in movement disorder patients.

In 1997, the FDA approved DBS for essential tremor and Parkinson-related tremor. More widespread cases of Parkinson's disease (PD) were approved in 2002, and in 2003, DBS was approved for dystonia on humanitarian grounds [9].

Although early promising research showed effectiveness and safety in treating patients with "primary" dystonia in both adults and children [10], during the past 20 years, surgical indications have expanded to include "secondary" dystonia, with varying and more distinct outcomes.

3. Mechanism of action

It is still unclear exactly what mechanism makes deep brain stimulation (DBS) effective. Deep brain stimulation (DBS) is believed to operate *via* a multimodal process, as suggested by a singular theory derived from several preclinical and clinical investigations aimed at elucidating its mechanisms [11]. A prominent perspective on this concept posits that the therapeutic effects of DBS arise from alterations in the activity of the target network [11, 12]. Consequently, identifying suitable target networks is essential for enhancing treatment outcomes [13], reinforcing the notion that DBS is classified as a form of network therapy.

4. Target selection

The globus pallidus internus (GPi) is currently the predominant target chosen for deep brain stimulation (DBS) therapy in CP and was initially documented in the treatment of dystonia [10]. Pallidal stimulation is extensively utilized in neuromodulation therapy for dyskinetic disorders, mostly due to its effectiveness in improving voluntary movements [14]. The majority of neurons in the globus pallidus are GABAergic [15]. The posteroventral GPi has become the specific target selected for the surgical treatment of most types of dystonia, including dystonia secondary to CP (**Figure 1**) [14].

Less often, other targets, such as the subthalamic nucleus (STN) [16] and particular thalamic regions, such as the ventral intermediate nucleus (Vim), ventral oral anterior (Voa), and ventral oral posterior (Vop) [17], have been reported to be effective in treating dystonia linked to cerebral palsy (**Figure 2**). In addition, deep brain stimulation of the dentate nuclei of the cerebellum in patients with CP appears to be safe and demonstrates initial signs of clinical benefit [18]. Currently, limited research on multitarget DBS has been documented in patients with CP [19].

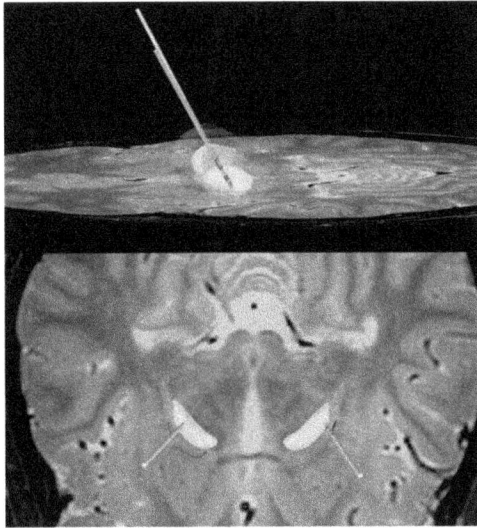

Figure 1.
Bilateral placement of DBS leads in the globus pallidus internus (GPi) in a patient with dystonic cerebral palsy.

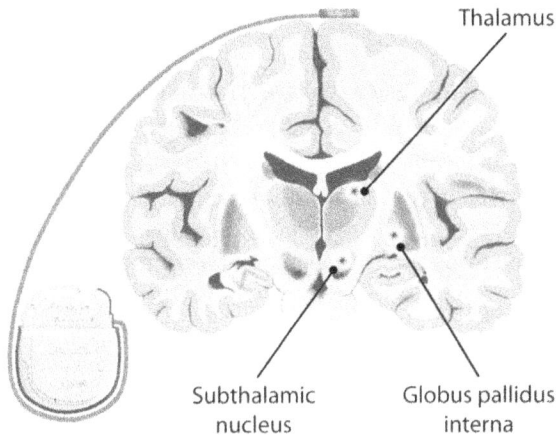

Figure 2.
Main DBS targets reported in cerebral palsy-related dystonia.

5. DBS surgery

DBS implantation is considered a stereotaxic neurosurgery procedure. Frame-based stereotaxis employs a rigid frame fixed to the skull. Before surgery, detailed imaging investigations, such as magnetic resonance imaging (MRI) and computed tomography (CT), are performed to identify precise target locations in the brain. During the procedure, a neurophysiological confirmation of the correct target can be done with microelectrode recording. Once the target is confirmed, permanent electrodes are inserted, successful placement is supported by testing electrical impedances, and side effects are assessed by test stimulation. Final electrode position can be determined with a postoperative CT scan; the scan can be overlaid on the preoperative MRI to confirm placement. Postoperative CT also allows exclusion of

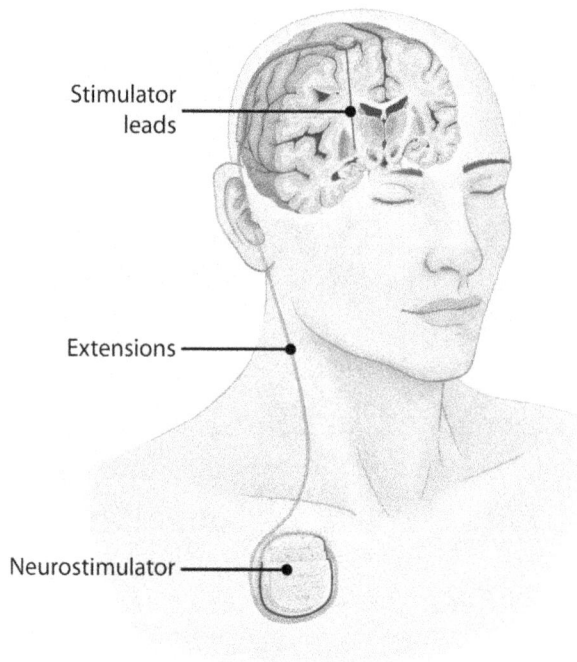

Figure 3.
Schematic representation of the components of a Deep Brain Stimulation (DBS) system.

hemorrhage. After the electrode implantation, they are connected to a pulse generator, which is usually placed in the chest; the generator implantation procedure and attachment to the connectors in the scalp *via* subcutaneously tunneled extension leads can be performed at the same time as permanent lead implantation, or in a separate procedure (**Figure 3**).

6. Programming

No defined guidelines exist for the postoperative therapy of patients with CP dystonia, especially regarding programming.

In programming DBS, four characteristics must be addressed for all patients: electrode configuration (contacts), amplitude, pulse width, and frequency (**Figure 4**) [20]. Programming regimens differ based on the clinician's expertise and patients' responses, with amplitudes from 1.0 to 6.5 V, pulse widths from 60 to 240 μs, and frequencies from 30 to 185 Hz [20]. The frequency of each programming session depends on the patient's answers, clinical assessments, and the particular requirements associated with their condition. Consistent follow-up evaluations are crucial for achieving optimal therapeutic results.

7. Efficacy for dystonia

The Burke-Fahn-Marsden Dystonia Rating Scale (BFMDRS) [21] is the predominant instrument for evaluating the severity of dystonia. It has been employed by

Pulse width (μs)
Duration of each stimulus

Amplitude
(Volts or miliamps)
Intensity of stimulation

Rate (Hz)
Number of pulses per second

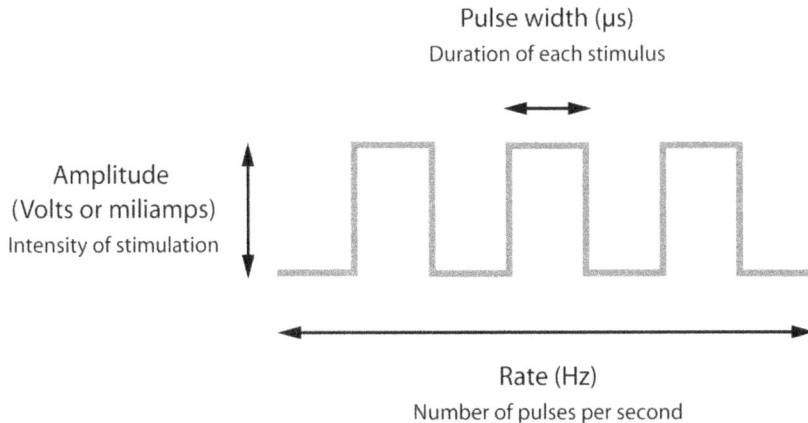

Figure 4.
Parameters to define during DBS programming.

numerous physicians and researchers to assess the therapeutic outcomes of DBS in cases of severe dystonia [22–24], including dystonia secondary to CP [6, 17, 22]. The BFMDRS consists of two clinician-assessed subscales: a movement subscale (MS), derived from patient evaluation, and a disability subscale (DS), based on the patient's self-reported difficulty in everyday activities. The BFMDRS has exhibited strong internal consistency, inter-rater reliability, and responsiveness in therapy investigations [25].

In contrast to the evident enhancement shown in Parkinson's disease, essential tremor, or primary dystonia, deep brain stimulation in secondary dystonia frequently yields advantages that are challenging to discern or measure [1, 22, 26].

In dystonia secondary to cerebral palsy, most research on Gpi DBS reveals a reduction in dystonia severity; however, clinical efficacy studies show highly variable results.

Elia et al. performed a literature review evaluating the efficacy of deep brain stimulation (DBS) for dystonia in individuals with cerebral palsy (CP), analyzing 124 patients across 12 trials published between 2009 and 2017. The review consistently indicated a decrease in motor symptoms of dystonia in all studies utilizing bilateral globus pallidus internus (GPi) DBS. Furthermore, a wide range of improvements in dystonia among CP patients was noted, with enhancements varying from a minimal 1.2% improvement in movement, as assessed by the Burke-Fahn-Marsden Dystonia Rating Scale (BFMDRS), to a substantial reduction in dystonia severity of up to 49.5% [20].

Furthermore, Koy et al. conducted a meta-analysis. Twenty publications involving 68 patients with cerebral palsy who had deep brain stimulation were evaluated using the Burke-Fahn-Marsden Dystonia Rating Scale. The majority of the articles were case reports, indicating significant heterogeneity in scores and follow-up duration. They reported a mean improvement of 23.6% (P < .001) in the movement scale and a mean improvement of 9.2% (P < .001) in the disability score on the Burke-Fahn-Marsden Dystonia Rating Scale at a median follow-up of 12 months. A substantial negative connection existed between the severity of dystonia and clinical outcomes (P < .05) [6].

In a separate recent study, Koy demonstrated that long-term DBS in pediatric patients with CP could have positive effects lasting up to 36 months. Motor improvement may not manifest within the initial postoperative year, indicating a possible but postponed impact of DBS on hyperkinetic movements [7].

The variability in these reported responses is mainly based on the fact that the studies conducted to date are quite heterogeneous and include patients with different severities of dystonia, variable ages, different causes of cerebral palsy, and different follow-up times [6, 17, 22, 27].

Several clinical factors have been associated with improved outcomes: reduced disease duration, younger surgical age, increased irregular intraoperative GPi micro-electrode firing frequency, and the absence of permanent skeletal abnormalities may act as favorable prognostic indicators for the therapeutic efficacy of DBS [28–31]. Conversely, cerebral lesions, dystonia severity, and associated spasticity may hinder therapeutic response [6, 31–33]; nevertheless, no set eligibility criteria currently exist.

Interesting, in cerebral palsy patients undergoing deep brain stimulation, even in the absence of apparent changes in motor symptoms or motor score improvement, patients frequently report enhanced ease of movement, more frequent and prolonged episodes of relaxation, and improved capacity to execute certain motor tasks [34].

8. Efficacy for other symptoms

Several studies indicate beneficial effects of DBS in pain perception, comfort, and particularly on overall quality of life [22, 35–37], even in patients where motor improvement measured by the BFMDRS scale is not evident [36]. Additionally, some studies have suggested improvements in speech and swallowing [8, 32], however, additional research is required to ascertain the actual impact of DBS on these specific issues.

Reports indicate that DBS may enhance several facets of psychological aspects, particularly with respect to interpersonal sensitivity, depression, paranoid ideation, and psychotic symptoms [22]. A cohort study examining children with dyskinetic cerebral palsy revealed that perceptual reasoning, improved post-DBS treatment, although overall cognitive function remained the same [15, 38].

The extent of benefit of DBS for non-motor symptoms remains ambiguous; the few studies conducted to date vary in the measured variables used to assess improvement in these symptoms. More prospective and homogeneous studies are needed on this topic.

9. Risks of DBS

Deep brain stimulation (DBS) surgery in CP patients, although invasive, frequently exhibits minimal complication rates. Adverse effects may be transitory, persistent, occur during surgical interventions, be associated with devices, or generated by stimulation, such dysarthria, paraesthesia, or loss of balance [39]. The primary adverse effects include infection, cerebral bleeding, electrode displacement, and hardware malfunctions [39]. The complication rate in pediatric patients undergoing DBS appears to be elevated compared to adult patients with ET or Parkinson's disease receiving DBS, particularly in those under the age of 10 [31]. This can be elucidated by the fact that patients receiving DBS at a young age typically present with Gross Motor Function Classification System (GMFCS) levels 4 or 5, indicating significant physical impairment accompanied by distracting symptoms such as immobility, sleep disturbances, and feeding difficulties, which contribute to malnourishment and diminished immunity, thereby increasing the likelihood of complications [31, 40].

In general, few significant surgical consequences have been documented for DBS treatment in cerebral palsy or other dystonic conditions. Numerous studies have suggested that DBS therapy is advantageous for CP patients.

10. Conclusions and future considerations

Despite the fact that the results of DBS in cerebral palsy are less consistent than in patients with monogenetic dystonia, DBS is considered a safe and effective treatment in patients with CP. The significant variation in results in this group of patients underscores the necessity for careful candidate selection for this intervention. Several critical characteristics, including severe and debilitating dystonia without significant underlying neurological diseases like spasticity or ataxia, are associated with improved results. Nevertheless, further investigation is necessary to clarify the influence of factors such as age at onset, duration of symptoms, and the patient's age during surgery.

Extensive, long-term, multicenter clinical trials could improve our comprehension of this neurosurgical intervention for patients with cerebral palsy by determining clinical determinants of positive results. Furthermore, it is crucial to consider improvements in the quality of life of patients and their caregivers, which may be more significant than the motor improvements achieved through this intervention.

Author details

Daniela Munoz-Chesta[1,2]* and Mónica Troncoso-Schifferli[1]

1 Department of Pediatric Neurology, San Borja Arriaran Hospital, University of Chile, Santiago, Chile

2 Department of Neurology, Neuroscience Center, Clinica Universidad de los Andes, Santiago, Chile

*Address all correspondence to: danielamch@gmail.com

IntechOpen

References

[1] Lin JP, Lumsden DE, Gimeno H, Kaminska M. The impact and prognosis for dystonia in childhood including dystonic cerebral palsy: A clinical and demographic tertiary cohort study. Journal of Neurology, Neurosurgery, and Psychiatry. 2014;**85**(11):1239-1244

[2] Rice J, Skuza P, Baker F, Russo R, Fehlings D. Identification and measurement of dystonia in cerebral palsy. Developmental Medicine and Child Neurology. 2017;**59**(12):1249-1255

[3] Albanese A, Bhatia K, Bressman SB, DeLong MR, Fahn S, Fung VSC, et al. Phenomenology and classification of dystonia: A consensus update: Dystonia: Phenomenology and classification. Movement Disorders. 2013;**28**(7):863-873

[4] Monbaliu E, Himmelmann K, Lin JP, Ortibus E, Bonouvrié L, Feys H, et al. Clinical presentation and management of dyskinetic cerebral palsy. Lancet Neurology. 2017;**16**(9):741-749

[5] Fehlings D, Agnew B, Gimeno H, Harvey A, Himmelmann K, Lin JP, et al. Pharmacological and neurosurgical management of cerebral palsy and dystonia: Clinical practice guideline update. Developmental Medicine and Child Neurology. 2024;**66**(9):1133-1147

[6] Koy A, Hellmich M, Pauls KAM, Marks W, Lin JP, Fricke O, et al. Effects of deep brain stimulation in dyskinetic cerebral palsy: A meta-analysis: Deep Brain Stimulation And Cerebral Palsy. Movement Disorders. 2013;**28**(5):647-654

[7] Koy A, Kühn AA, Schiller P, Huebl J, Schneider GH, Eckenweiler M, et al. Long-term follow-up of pediatric patients with dyskinetic cerebral palsy and deep brain stimulation. Movement Disorders. 2023;**38**(9):1736-1742

[8] Keen JR, Przekop A, Olaya JE, Zouros A, Hsu FPK. Deep brain stimulation for the treatment of childhood dystonic cerebral palsy. Journal of Neurosurgery. Pediatrics. 2014;**14**(6):585-593

[9] Gardner J. A history of deep brain stimulation: Technological innovation and the role of clinical assessment tools. Social Studies of Science. 2013;**43**(5):707-728

[10] Coubes P, Roubertie A, Vayssiere N, Hemm S, Echenne B. Treatment of DYT1-generalised dystonia by stimulation of the internal globus pallidus. The Lancet. 2000;**355**(9222):2220-2221

[11] Neumann WJ, Steiner LA, Milosevic L. Neurophysiological mechanisms of deep brain stimulation across spatiotemporal resolutions. Brain. 2023;**146**(11):4456-4468

[12] Sobesky L, Goede L, Odekerken VJJ, Wang Q, Li N, Neudorfer C, et al. Subthalamic and pallidal deep brain stimulation: Are we modulating the same network? Brain. 2022;**145**(1):251-262

[13] Sandoval-Pistorius SS, Hacker ML, Waters AC, Wang J, Provenza NR, de Hemptinne C, et al. Advances in deep brain stimulation: From mechanisms to applications. The Journal of Neuroscience. 2023;**43**(45):7575-7586

[14] Cif L, Hariz M. Seventy years of pallidotomy for movement disorders. Movement Disorders. 2017;**32**(7):972-982

[15] Jiang H, Wang R, Zheng Z, Zhu J. Deep brain stimulation for the treatment

of cerebral palsy: A review. Brain Science Advances. 2020;**6**(1):20-29

[16] Starr PA, Markun LC, Larson PS, Volz MM, Martin AJ, Ostrem JL. Interventional MRI–guided deep brain stimulation in pediatric dystonia: First experience with the ClearPoint system: Clinical article. Journal of Neurosurgery. Pediatrics. 2014;**14**(4):400-408

[17] Wolf ME, Blahak C, Saryyeva A, Schrader C, Krauss JK. Deep brain stimulation for dystonia-choreoathetosis in cerebral palsy: Pallidal versus thalamic stimulation. Parkinsonism & Related Disorders. 2019;**63**:209-212

[18] Cajigas I, Morrison MA, Luciano MS, Starr PA. Cerebellar deep brain stimulation for the treatment of movement disorders in cerebral palsy. Journal of Neurosurgery. 2023;**139**(3):605-614

[19] Goel A, Narayan SK, Sugumaran R. Hemiplegic cerebral palsy complicated by acute hemidystonia in adulthood. Neurology Clinical Practice. 2021;**11**(5):e736-e739

[20] Elia AE, Bagella CF, Ferré F, Zorzi G, Calandrella D, Romito LM. Deep brain stimulation for dystonia due to cerebral palsy: A review. European Journal of Paediatric Neurology. 2018;**22**(2):308-315

[21] Burke RE, Fahn S, Marsden CD, Bressman SB, Moskowitz C, Friedman J. Validity and reliability of a rating scale for the primary torsion dystonias. Neurology. 1985;**35**(1):73-73

[22] Vidailhet M, Yelnik J, Lagrange C, Fraix V, Grabli D, Thobois S, et al. Bilateral pallidal deep brain stimulation for the treatment of patients with dystonia-choreoathetosis cerebral palsy: A prospective pilot study. Lancet Neurology. 2009;**8**(8):709-717

[23] Vidailhet M, Vercueil L, Houeto JL, Krystkowiak P, Lagrange C, Yelnik J, et al. Bilateral, pallidal, deep-brain stimulation in primary generalised dystonia: A prospective 3 year follow-up study. Lancet Neurology. 2007;**6**(3):223-229

[24] Holloway KL, Baron MS, Brown R, Cifu DX, Carne W, Ramakrishnan V. Deep brain stimulation for dystonia: A meta-analysis. Neuromodulation: Technology at the Neural Interface. 2006;**9**(4):253-261

[25] Comella CL, Leurgans S, Wuu J, Stebbins GT, Chmura T, The Dystonia Study Group. Rating scales for dystonia: A multicenter assessment. Movement Disorders. 2003;**18**(3):303-312

[26] Marks W, Bailey L, Sanger TD. PEDiDBS: The pediatric international deep brain stimulation registry project. European Journal of Paediatric Neurology. 2017;**21**(1):218-222

[27] Nunta-aree S, Nimmannitya P, Sitthinamsuwan B, Pisarnpong A, Boonyapisit K. Clinical outcome of pallidal deep brain stimulation for various types of dystonia. Journal of the Medical Association of Thailand. 2017;**100**(Suppl. 3):S103-S110

[28] Isaias IU, Volkmann J, Kupsch A, Burgunder JM, Ostrem JL, Alterman RL, et al. Factors predicting protracted improvement after pallidal DBS for primary dystonia: The role of age and disease duration. Journal of Neurology. 2011;**258**(8):1469-1476

[29] Andrews C, Aviles-Olmos I, Hariz M, Foltynie T. Which patients with dystonia benefit from deep brain stimulation? A metaregression of individual patient outcomes. Journal of Neurology, Neurosurgery, and Psychiatry. 2010;**81**(12):1383-1389

[30] Lumsden DE, Kaminska M, Gimeno H, Tustin K, Baker L, Perides S, et al. Proportion of life lived with dystonia inversely correlates with response to pallidal deep brain stimulation in both primary and secondary childhood dystonia. Developmental Medicine and Child Neurology. 2013;**55**(6):567-574

[31] Koy A, Timmermann L. Deep brain stimulation in cerebral palsy: Challenges and opportunities. European Journal of Paediatric Neurology. 2017;**21**(1):118-121

[32] Romito LM, Zorzi G, Marras CE, Franzini A, Nardocci N, Albanese A. Pallidal stimulation for acquired dystonia due to cerebral palsy: Beyond 5 years. European Journal of Neurology. 2015;**22**(3):426-e32

[33] Cif L. Deep brain stimulation in dystonic cerebral palsy: For whom and for what? European Journal of Neurology. 2015;**22**(3):423-425

[34] Sanger TD. Deep brain stimulation for cerebral palsy: Where are we now? Developmental Medicine and Child Neurology. 2020;**62**(1):28-33

[35] Aihemaitiniyazi A, Zhang H, Hu Y, Li T, Liu C. Quality of life outcomes after deep brain stimulation in acquired dystonia: A systematic review and meta-analysis. Neurological Sciences. 2024;**45**(2):467-476

[36] Gimeno H, Tustin K, Selway R, Lin JP. Beyond the Burke–Fahn–Marsden Dystonia Rating Scale: Deep brain stimulation in childhood secondary dystonia. European Journal of Paediatric Neurology. 2012;**16**(5):501-508

[37] Koy A, Kühn AA, Huebl J, Schneider G, Riesen AK, Eckenweiler M, et al. Quality of life after deep brain stimulation of pediatric patients with dyskinetic cerebral palsy: A prospective, single-arm, multicenter study with a subsequent randomized double-blind crossover (STIM-CP). Movement Disorders. 2022;**37**(4):799-811

[38] Owen T, Gimeno H, Selway R, Lin JP. Cognitive function in children with primary dystonia before and after deep brain stimulation. European Journal of Paediatric Neurology. 2015;**19**(1):48-55

[39] Fenoy AJ, Simpson RK. Risks of common complications in deep brain stimulation surgery: Management and avoidance: Clinical article. Journal of Neurosurgery. 2014;**120**(1):132-139

[40] Air EL, Starr PA. Deep brain stimulation in children: Experience and technical pearls. Journal of Neurosurgery. 2011;**8**:9

Chapter 2

Neurosurgical Management of Spasticity

Ziyad Makoshi

Abstract

Cerebral palsy is the most common cause of motor disability in children. Its associated movements disorders are variable, but spasticity is the most common type identified on clinical assessment. Spasticity can involve any or all of the extremities, and its presence can lead to a negative impact on function and quality of life. Several treatments, both medical and surgical have been developed over the years to help relieve spasticity and improve function. These are often used in combination based on recommendations from a multidisciplinary team assessment to what best suits a particular individual. Neurosurgery interventions for spasticity include baclofen pump placement and selective dorsal rhizotomies.

Keywords: spasticity, rhizotomy, baclofen, cerebral palsy, GMFCS

1. Introduction

The ability to move our limbs with ease allows us to engage in a multitude of activities and careers. A small increase in muscle tone (hypertonia) or hyperkinetic movements (e.g., dystonia) can lead to difficulties with everyday tasks, especially in children, including running, playing, or climbing stairs. It is important to recognize that these movement disorders can occur for many reasons, and there are several types that require an accurate diagnosis and do not always occur in isolation. The Task Force on Childhood Motor Disorders provides a consensus definition on three common types; spasticity, rigidity, and dystonia [1].

Spasticity is identified by resistance to passive movement across a joint, and resistance increases with the speed of movement, i.e., so-called "velocity-dependent hypertonia." Rigidity is different in that the hypertonia is present in both passive and active movement similar at any speed, and involves both agonist and antagonist muscles evident by immediate resistance with reversal in the direction of movement. Dystonia is recognized by the presence of involuntary sustained or intermittent muscle contractions causing twisting and repetitive movements, abnormal postures, or both and occurs during voluntary (active) movement [1]. Identifying and distinguishing the presence of one or more of these on clinical exam is important in the management of individuals with movement disorders.

This distinction is not always easy in children or individuals who cannot cooperate with the examiner. Hypotonia can sometimes be mistaken with hypertonia if the child actively resists the examiner during perceived "passive" range of motion. In these circumstances, patience and timing when the child is distracted or relaxed may offer a more reliable assessment, and asking the care giver about their experience during passive movement of the limb when caring for the child and observations when the child is active can be a hint to the nature of the muscle tone. The presence of fixed contractures is another limitation to the examination of tone and should be taken into consideration.

When considering the cause of hypertonia in particular, any injury along the central nervous system (CNS) can lead to a disruption in the balanced excitatory-inhibitory control on downstream pathways, with a net loss of inhibitory control leading to hyperexcitability. This explanation is overly simplistic and the pathways responsible for these movement disorders are better reviewed elsewhere [2]. However, this illustrates that many possible causes of hypertonia exist, including trauma (e.g., traumatic brain or spinal cord injury, iatrogenic), demyelination (e.g., multiple sclerosis), stroke (e.g., hemorrhagic or ischemic), CNS infections (e.g., congenital or post-natal), certain metabolic and genetic disorders, and perinatal CNS injury [3]. Injury to the developing brain causing a clinical manifestation as the child grows has been broadly grouped under the umbrella term cerebral palsy (CP).

2. Cerebral palsy: Historical perspective and current definitions

Debate on the causes of hemiplegia were presented early in the 1800s based on post-mortem pathology reports describing contralateral atrophy of the brain in hemiplegic individuals [4]. In the mid-1800s, an orthopedic surgeon by the name of William Little, with a keen interest in orthopedic foot deformities[1] and through meticulous history taking, clinical examination, and documentation discovered a possible correlation between perinatal injury and prematurity with later development of spasticity and movement disorders among other clinical manifestations [5]. His work and lectures on the topic lead to the eponymous referral by others as "Little's disease" [6]. The term cerebral palsy was soon introduced by Sir William Osler in his 1889 publication "The Cerebral Palsies of Children" and his classification by distribution and location is still used today in a modified fashion [7]. By the end of the nineteenth century, Sigmund Freud had published several writings on CP making major contribution in the neuropathology of the disease and dividing the etiology into congenital, perinatally acquired, and postnatally acquired [8]. Their contributions, among many others, led to thousands of publications on the topic in the early twentieth century [9].

Many definitions of CP with various iterations and updates have occurred since then [10, 11]. More recently, the Surveillance of Cerebral Palsy in Europe (SCPE) network recommended that centers continue to use their definition of choice, but that it include five main components: "CP is a group of disorders i.e. it is an umbrella term; it is permanent but not unchanging; it involves a disorder of movement and/or posture and of motor function; it is due to a non-progressive interference/lesion/abnormality; this interference/lesion/abnormality is in the developing/immature brain" [12]. In 2005, the Executive Committee for the Definition of Cerebral Palsy offered the following: "[CP] describes a group of disorders of the development of movement and posture, causing activity limitation, that are attributed to non-progressive disturbances that occurred in the developing fetal or infant

---

[1] This should come as no surprise as he too suffered from club foot after contracting poliomyelitis and had another surgeon perform a tendon release on him with much relief.

brain. The motor disorders of cerebral palsy are often accompanied by disturbances of sensation, cognition, communication, perception, and/or behavior, and/or by a seizure disorder" [13]. These broad definitions reflect the many issues an individual with CP may encounter, and the need for a multidisciplinary approach to improve functionality and quality of life.

3. Cerebral palsy and spasticity: Classification and assessment scales

The incidence of CP appears to be around 2–3 per 1000 live births in developed countries [12], but shows wider variability and higher numbers in developing countries [14–16]. It is almost certain that health care provides will encounter at least one patient in their practice with CP. Various classification schemes exit based on several domains proposed by the American Academy for Cerebral Palsy, of which three have been recommended clinicians use; based on motor symptoms, topographical involvement, or etiology [17]. The SCPE classifies CP by motor symptoms into spastic (unilateral or bilateral), dyskinetic (dystonic or choreo-athetotic), ataxic, and non-classifiable [12]. The Executive Committee for the Definition of Cerebral Palsy—recognizing the limitations in prior classifications, proposed four main components: motor abnormalities (i.e., the tone, type of movement disorder, and functional motor abilities), associated impairments (i.e., non-motor neurodevelopmental, sensory, or cognitive problems), anatomical and radiological findings, causation and timing (if known). To help provide best practice recommendations for baclofen treatment, an expert panel critically reviewed the definition of spasticity used above given its constraint and proposed the following: "[spasticity is] disordered sensori-motor control, resulting from an upper motor neuron lesion, presenting as intermittent or sustained involuntary activation of muscles," thereby providing a more general definition for use in clinical practice [18].

Spasticity is by the far the most common motor manifestation of CP (~85%) and spastic diplegia the most common subtype (50–60%) [19]. Classifying spasticity shows some heterogeneity across centers [20], but a common and long standing approach is based on limb involvement into spastic hemiplegia, diplegia, and quadriplegia. In the pursuit of treating spasticity in individuals diagnosed with CP, the provider should be aware of some key points. It is important to note that classification is based on the predominant motor type, but that mixed types (e.g., spastic-dyskinetic) are not uncommon [21]. Muscle tone appears to increase during the first 4 to 5 years of life with some decrease thereafter until early teenage years with no significant change thereafter [22–24]. While gross motor functional status appears to peak around 6 to 7 years of age [25, 26], in those more severely affected it may occur much earlier [27] and with some decline thereafter into early adulthood [26].

Several measures have been developed for the assessment of spasticity and motor function to categorize severity, functional status, response to therapy, and to standardize reporting. In 1964, during his work with individuals suffering from multiple sclerosis, Bryan Ashworth described the Ashworth scale to grade spasticity [28]. This 5 point scale, from 0 to 4, was modified in 1987 by adding a 1+ description to increase sensitivity (**Table 1**) [29]. To assess changes over time or with intervention, the gross motor function measure (GMFM) was developed in 1989 [30], which includes two versions and is now in its third edition [31]. The GMFM-88 is the original 88-item measure, includes five domains, and can be used for children with more complex disability including those requiring mobility aids. Item are scored 0 to 3 and then

0	No increase in muscle tone
1	Slight increase in muscle tone, manifested by a catch and release or by minimal resistance at the end of the range of motion when the affected part/s is/are moved in flexion or extension.
1+	Slight increase in muscle tone, manifested by a catch, followed by minimal resistance throughout the remainder (less than half) of the ROM.
2	More marked increase in muscle tone through most of the ROM, but affected part(s) easily moved.
3	Considerable increase in muscle tone, passive movement difficult.
4	Affected part(s) rigid in flexion or extension

Table 1.
Modified Ashworth Scale for spasticity grading [29].

summed to calculate raw and percent scores for each domain; percent scores are then averaged to obtain an overall total score. In an effort to grade the functional status in children across different age groups, the gross motor classification system (GMFCS) was published in 1997 and includes levels 1 and 2 for those independently ambulatory, level 3 if assistance is required, and levels 4 and 5 whom are non-ambulatory [32]. The GMFM-66 is a 66 item subset of the original GMFM-88 that requires less time, and can be used to follow change over time or to compare patterns of change. A program is used to calculate a score from 0 to 100 and based on the child's GMFCS level and age, the score can then be plotted on the corresponding motor growth curve to help predict likely motor development. Familiarity with these assessment tools provides the reader with the necessary knowledge to interpret clinical reports and studies as will be used here.

4. Spasticity: Neurosurgical management—Baclofen pumps

ɣ-Aminobutyric acid, or GABA, is the major inhibitory neurotransmitter in the CNS [33]. The receptor subtype involved in spasticity is $GABA_B$ [34], however, GABA which was first synthesized in 1883[2] is a poor therapeutic option as it does not cross the blood brain barrier (BBB) [35]. It wasn't until 1962, that β-(4-chlorophenyl)-ɣ-aminobutyric acid (β-(4-chlorophenyl)-GABA), later to be known as baclofen, was first synthesized and was able to penetrate the BBB [36]. Originally meant to treat epilepsy, its clinical use for spasticity became quickly apparent and it was approved by the FDA for this use in 1977 (interestingly, this was several years before the $GABA_B$ receptor it worked on was discovered). Oral baclofen was not without its limitations; including multiple dose requirements per day with only a small portion crossing the BBB [36], and its central depression effects (sedation, confusion, somnolence) [37]. To minimize these effect and optimize its muscle relaxant potential, intrathecal baclofen was approved by the FDA in 1992 for spasticity of spinal origin and in 1996 for spasticity of cerebral origin. It is available under several trade names including Lioresal (oral), Gablofen (injectable), Kemstro (disenegrating formulation), Lioresal intrathecal and Ozobax (oral solution).

---

[2] Although it was later in the 1950s and 1960s that it was demonstrated to exist in mammalian CNS and its inhibitory action on neuronal activity.

4.1 Mechanism

Baclofen works on $GABA_B$ receptors located in the cortex and spine, its activation leads to hyperpolarization of the neuron, which leads to inhibition of neurotransmitter release, thereby blocking mono- and polysynaptic reflexes in the spine that mediate spasticity resulting in reduced muscle tone [38]. Dosing is in micrograms rather than milligrams for oral dosing (100th of the dose), reaching four times the concentration of an oral route in the cerebrospinal fluid (CSF) [39], faster acting within 30 to 60 minutes [40], with maximum effect around 4 hours after bolus injection and gone by 8–10 hours [41]. While intrathecal infusion onset of action occurs at 6–8 hours and reaches peak effect at 24–48 hours, with a half-life of approximately 5 hours [42]. Patients often do not require multiple other medications for spasticity as can be needed for oral baclofen. A programable baclofen pump has been developed by several manufactures. The basic components of the pump include a programmable reservoir that has a port for transcutaneous filling of the pump with baclofen, a catheter connected to the pump through a port, often with a port access to allow CSF aspiration, and a catheter that is placed within the intradural space to allow delivery of the drug directly into the CSF. The average life of a programmable baclofen pump is approximately 6 years but varies considerably and at this time requires surgical replacement when the battery is near depletion.

4.2 Indications

Indications for baclofen pump consideration include severe spasticity that has failed medical management (i.e., poor response, intolerance, side effects). Severe spasticity has been considered an Ashworth score ≥ 3, however, some have argued that "severe" should apply to any individual severely affected by spasticity in a negative manner in regard to their functionality, care, or quality of life [43]. Most providers will then proceed with a trial of intrathecal baclofen (25–100 μg based on weight and response) and assess the patient over several hours for any improvement in tone (ideally an improvement of 2 or more points on the Ashworth scale) and sometimes function [44, 45]. Several benefits exist with this approach including identifying a response dose, tolerability, and expectations, as well as serving as a basis for daily dose initiation once the pump is implanted (generally double the positive trial dose per day). Others argue that a trial may not accurately predict long term benefits in all patients and requires a separate procedure [44], and proceeding with placement can be for those meeting clinical criteria. For those with spastic diplegia, selective dorsal rhizotomy can be considered.

4.3 Evidence

The work by Dralle et al. in the 1980s and Albright et al. in 1991 showing the benefit in tone reduction of intrathecal baclofen injection compared to placebo in individuals with CP, paved the way for its use in clinical practice and formed the basis for trial dosing still used today [46–48]. A Cochrane review included mostly intrathecal trial studies and concluded that a significant improvement in spasticity was evident short term but could not comment on long term results [49]. The work by Albright and colleagues during the 1990s continued to mount evidence for the benefits of baclofen pump placement in tone reduction for individuals with CP suffering from spasticity [50–52]. Longer term follow up studies confirmed ongoing improvement in tone reduction and quality of life scores [53–55]. It is important to note that the majority of these individuals had spastic diplegia or spastic quadriplegia involvement. A recent meta-analysis and system review found that intrathecal baclofen treatment leads to a significant improvement in tone reduction and likely some motor function improvement in certain individuals, however the rate of complications was 40% and this will be discussed in more detail below [56]. Clinical evidence of intrathecal baclofen use in various conditions has been well reviewed elsewhere [57, 58].

Two other considerations regarding the effects of baclofen pump placement are whether any changes in the rate of scoliosis progression or need for orthopedic surgery occurs. A recent meta-analysis on scoliosis progression found evidence that baclofen pump treatment may accelerate worsening of the curve [59], and perhaps the current state of evidence is best summed as baclofen pump placement may or may not effect development of scoliosis, but may contribute to its progression in individuals with pre-exiting scoliosis. In regard to the need for further orthopedic surgery, despite an early publication that it does decrease this rate [60], several studies thereafter suggest that it does not ultimately change the need for orthopedic surgery [61, 62]. Rather than this being a goal of baclofen pump placement, orthopedic surgery should be thought of as another component of managing individuals with spasticity especially once tone reduction is achieved and joint mobility remains limited due to contractions or muscle/tendon shortening and may be preventing further improvement in function.

Even if a baclofen pump is deemed to be a good option for the patient, certain patient related factors may increase the risk of complications so much so that a pump may be contraindicated. This includes body habitus, e.g., small size for pump placement (although prior tissue expander use has been described [63]), severe spinal deformity limiting the abdominal area for the pump to safely be implanted, malnutrition and low weight increasing the risk of skin breakdown. If all these factors align and this opens the door for discussing this option with patients and families, several considerations should be taken into account by the health care provider. The commitment, resources, and support needed to manage a baclofen pump program are paramount because pump malfunction or delayed refill/pump replacement can be life threatening. Any physician or centers that decide to provide this service to patients should consider the following:

- Establishing a multidisciplinary team for correct and accurate diagnosis of spasticity related conditions including CP, and to identify appropriate candidates,

- A clinic setting and provider(s) trained and able to monitor reservoir volume status and provide refills in a timely manner to avoid risk of baclofen withdrawal,

- A surgeon trained and competent in placement, management of complications, and replacement of baclofen pumps,

- An inpatient team (e.g., physiatrist) familiar with baclofen pump management and able to interrogate and investigate possible pump malfunction, and

- Hospitalist/intensivists familiar with baclofen withdrawal symptoms for early identification and immediate oral and intravenous medical management and close monitoring

4.4 Surgical technique and nuances

4.4.1 Planning

Best practice for surgical implantation is well described elsewhere [64], a brief description is presented here along with evidence of benefit/risk for each step where available. A detailed preoperative history and examination is paramount, the surgeon should be aware of prior surgeries that may impact positioning, incisions, and tunneling. These include prior ventricular peritoneal shunts (VPS) that may traverse the abdominal incision site, scoliosis surgery, and epilepsy surgery implants such as Vagus Nerve Stimulators that are affected by cautery.

4.4.2 Setup

The patient is positioned in the left lateral decubitus position (unless there is a clinical indication to place the pump on the left side, e.g., ileotomy, severe dextrocardia, VPS tubing) with the head supported toward anesthesia in a neutral position. The surgical bed should allow for the fluoroscopy machine to easily move across the torso during placement and advancement of the intrathecal catheter for appropriate and accurate positioning (although some centers place catheters based on preoperative measurements without routine intraoperative fluoroscopy [65]). The author uses this position for pump replacements as well to be prepared for any revision on the catheter side if ever needed without breaking sterility. An axillary roll is placed under the left (dependent) upper chest to prevent compression of the brachial artery and plexus. The hips and knees are gently flexed and all pressure points should be appropriately padded including between the knees and the dependent lateral aspect of the knee and ankle.

4.4.3 Incisions

Two incisions are marked, the first across the abdomen along the right subcostal space (the length slightly longer than the diameter of the pump being used which is selected based on patient weight, body habitus, and desired volume) and a second along the midline lumbar spine at L2–3 or L3–4 (**Figures 1** and **2**). Variations to this approach may be needed based on prior incisions or surgeries in the abdomen (e.g., laparotomy scars, feeding tubes) and if any concern, general surgery should be consulted for assistance. In regard to the lumbar incision, some prefer to place the incision off midline but there is a concern if the child requires spine surgery in the future for deformity which is not uncommon that a prior incision may be missed and vascular supply to the skin compromised. In a similar fashion, any prior spine surgery incisions should be taken into consideration during planning.

4.4.4 Preparation

The surgical sites are prepped and draped in a sterile fashion to allow access to the abdomen, right flank, and lumbar spine (**Figures 1** and **2**). Perioperative antibiotics and double gloving are recommended based on VPS data [66, 67]. The baclofen pump is programmed in its sterile container prior to opening it onto the sterile field, after which the reservoir is filled based on the pump size (volume) selected—if performing

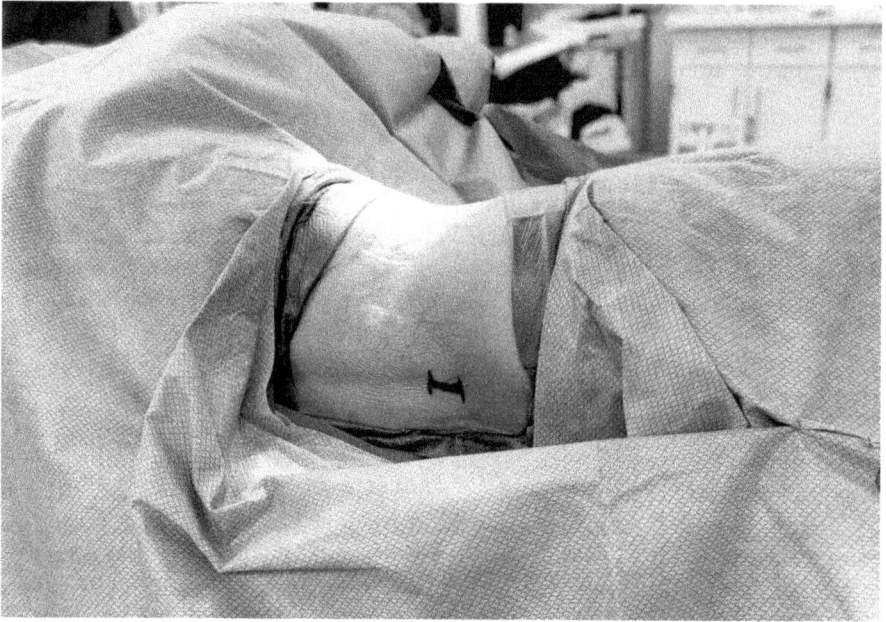

Figure 1.
Right decubitus positioning of a patient for baclofen pump placement. An L3–4 incision is marked. Appropriate padding of all pressure points and axillary roll is important to avoid any neurovascular compression.

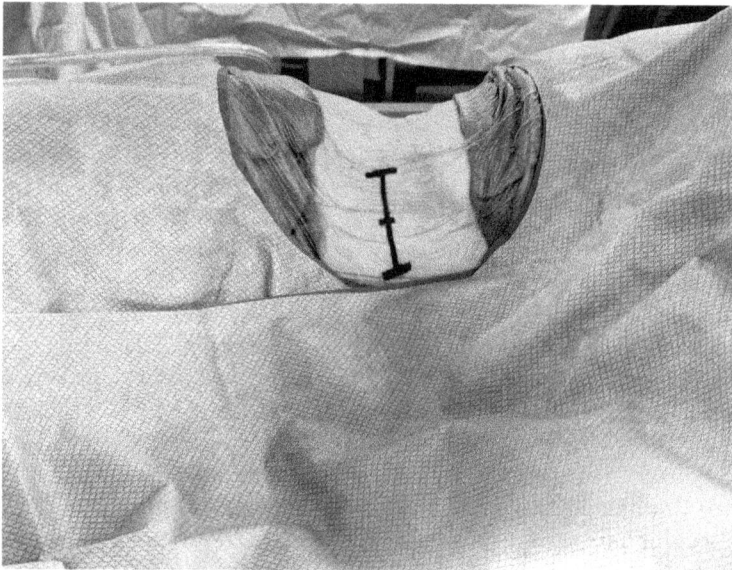

Figure 2.
Right subcostal abdominal incision measured to the size of the baclofen pump to be used.

the procedure for the first time, communication with the pharmacist to prepare baclofen for intrathecal use in the appropriate volume can save time and allow for more efficiency.

4.4.5 Surgical steps part 1 - spinal portion

Starting with the lumbar incision is recommended [68] as this is the part of the procedure most likely to encounter any problems. The lumbar incision is carried out in the interspinous space to the level of the fascia. The Tuohy needle is then placed under fluoroscopic guidance into the interspinous space one to two levels above to create some distance between the incision and the dural entry point using an off-midline entry—this is based on consensus recommendations rather than clinical data [68]. Tactile feedback and return of CSF along with correlated position on X-ray confirm entry in the intradural space (**Figure 3**). The catheter with the stylet in place is then passed under fluoroscopy guidance to the desired level (lower thoracic spine for spastic diplegia and upper thoracic spine for spastic tetraplegia or quadriplegia) (**Figure 4**).

4.4.6 Nuances for catheter placement

Resistance encountered during placement can be managed by gently rotating the catheter between the thumb and index finger and trying to slowly advance again (if caught on a nerve root or dentate ligament). If the catheter needs to be withdrawn for any reason, this should be done with the Tuohy needle to avoid tearing the catheter along the edge of the needle. The needle is then withdrawn with careful control of the catheter to avoid pull out and an anchor (often provided as part of the set) is passed along the catheter into the fascial opening and sutured in place to minimize risk of

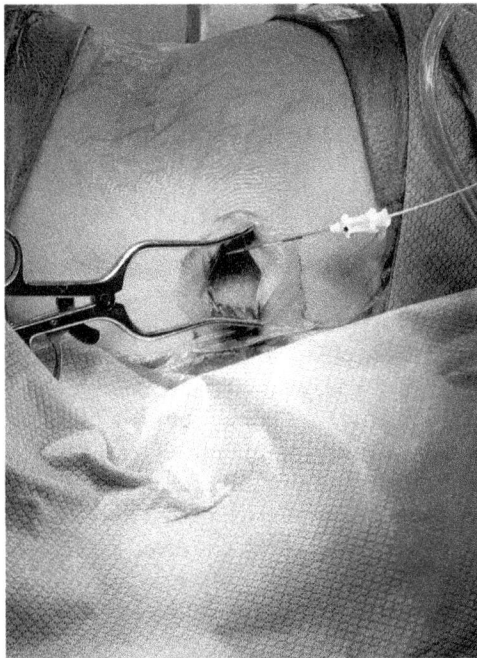

Figure 3.
Paramedian insertion of the spinal needle to pass the intrathecal catheter under fluoroscopy. Note the drop of CSF along the needle confirming entry into the thecal sac.

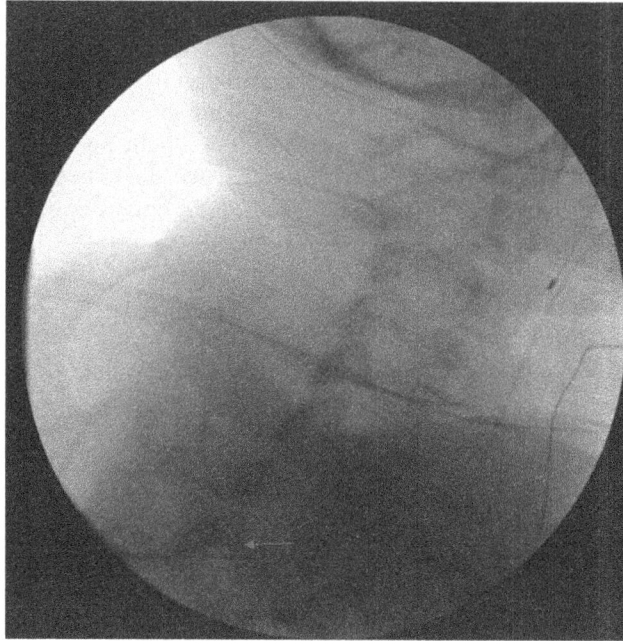

Figure 4.
Location of the catheter tip (blue arrow) during advancement under fluoroscopy to the desired level based on the indication for the baclofen pump.

out-migration of the catheter (**Figure 5**). CSF should be seen to be dripping from the distal end of the catheter during and the end of this part of the procedure to confirm patency (techniques in the absence of CSF flow have included contrast injection under fluoroscopy to document a myelogram [69], or a hemilaminectomy to confirm dural entry). Other options if lumbar access is not possible include cervical placement [70] and intraventricular placement [71].

4.4.7 Surgical steps part 2 - abdominal portion

The abdominal incision is opened and dissection carried down to fascia. Both subcutaneous and subfascial placement are described and each carry benefits and risks. For children under 50 pounds, a subfascial dissection should be considered to minimize risk of skin breakdown [72, 73], however risk of migration into the intra-peritoneal cavity has been reported [74]. Submuscular placement in older children and adults with very low weights has also been described [75]. The size of the pocket created should allow the baclofen pump to be placed deep enough without the edge of the device causing pressure on the incision. The distal catheter is then tunneled in the subcutaneous tissue across the right flank toward the abdominal incision and attached to the baclofen pump catheter through a connector (**Figure 6**).

4.4.8 Pump placement and closure

The pump is then placed into the pocket created in the abdomen and the reservoir port should be facing outward to allow refilling, and the catheter access port rotated away from the incision to allow aspiration without a needle passing close to the

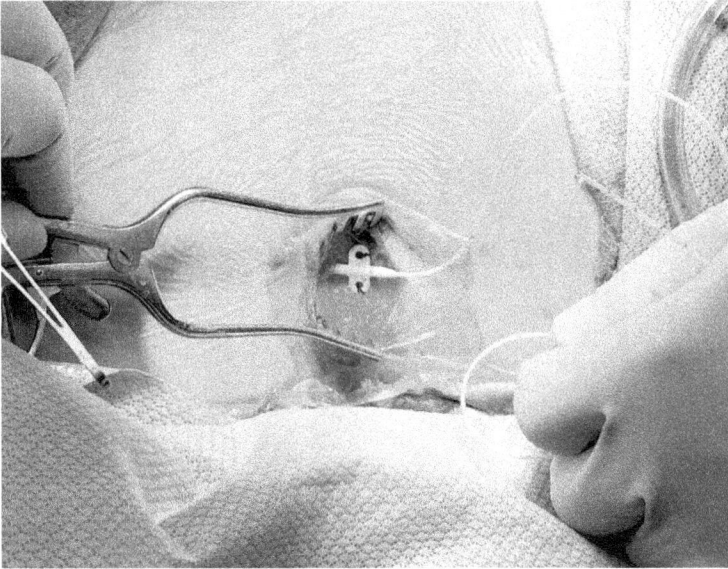

Figure 5.
Attachment of the anchor which serves to fill the hole within the fascia and minimize risk of a CSF leak, and suturing of the anchor to the fascia to minimize risk of migration of the catheter. Note the drop of CSF along the catheter confirming the trip is within the thecal sac.

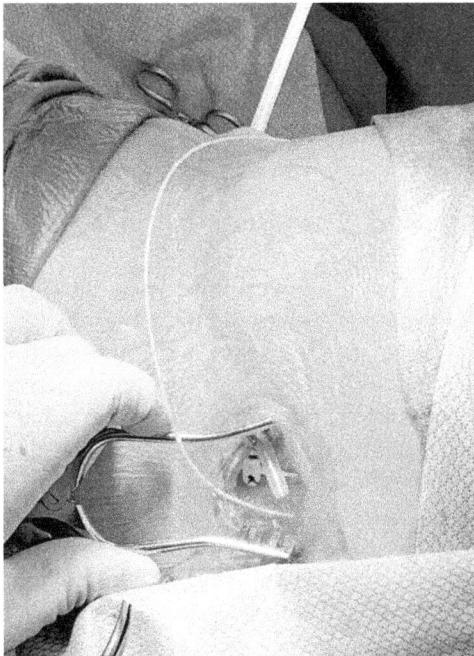

Figure 6.
Tunneling from the abdominal cavity to the spinal cavity to pass the catheter.

incision (**Figure 7**). The pump is then anchored in at least three of the suture loops to minimized risk of rotation. This is suspected when the reprogramming or refills are unsuccessful (other techniques to minimize the risk of rotation or flipping include

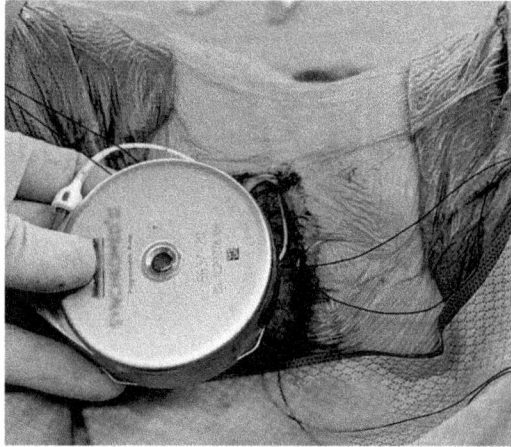

Figure 7.
Catheter port attached to the baclofen pump with the silk ties in place to minimize risk of rotation or flipping of the pump. Note positioning of the access port away from the incision to minimize risk of infection when access is needed percutaneously.

avoiding an oversized pocket size, and a sock placed over the pump to promote scarring down) [76]. Any excess catheter is tucked behind the pump in a relaxed loop to minimize risk of kinking or injury during revision. Aspiration of CSF from the access port prior to closure confirms patency of the system and should aspirate freely and with minimal resistance depending on the size of needle used. The use of topical antibiotics has been described by some to decrease the risk of surgical site infections [77]. It is important that good wound care be discussed with the patient and family during the healing process to minimize risk of surgical site complications and identify any wound issues early.

4.5 Complications, workup, and management

Complications unfortunately are not uncommon with baclofen pumps and patients and their families should be educated to monitor for signs and symptoms for early identification and treatment. The rate varies across studies, but it is estimated that 1 in 4 to 1 in 5 individuals will have a baclofen pump related complication. These complications are also more common in the pediatric age group than in adults [76, 78]. Complications can be thought of in two broad categories, potentially avoidable (patient selection and surgical technique related as was presented above) and system related, which can be further divided into catheter, pump, and cavity related issues (abdominal and intradural) and will be elaborated on here. Any individual with a suspected pump malfunction should have a thorough history and clinical exam completed and medically stabilized, if necessary, prior to proceeding with further investigations.

Catheter related complications appear to be the most common reason for pump malfunction in children and adults and tend to occur several months or years after surgery [65, 76, 79, 80]. These can include fracture, kinking, detachment, occlusion or migration (iatrogenic injury has also been seen with scoliosis surgery and placement of drains where the trocar cuts the catheter during tunneling). Signs and symptoms can either be a decrease in the effectiveness of the baclofen dose with poor response to dose increase if some baclofen is still making its way into the intradural space or acute baclofen withdrawal if minimal to no baclofen is being delivered. Identification of this issue will often require imaging: multiple view X-rays, fluoroscopy, and CT ± intra-thecal safe dye and radionucleotide studies are all options to investigate the entire length of the catheter for any leakage, increased resistance to injection, fracture, kinking, migration, or detachment [81]. The CSF access port should be tapped first to confirm patency, aspirate to rule out any CSF infection, and remove baclofen within the catheter prior to injection to avoid delivering an overdose during testing, if CSF cannot be aspirated then it is recommended not to proceed with any contrast studies [82]. Treatment involves surgical revision of the catheter. Microfractures can also occur and are difficult to diagnose as the workup may appear "normal" but the patient can exhibit intermittent signs of baclofen withdrawal [83]. Additionally, arachnoid adhesions around the catheter tip can form in long standing pumps and lead to intermittent alternating hyper- and hypotonia episodes based on random delivery of baclofen into the intradural space through the adhesions. Therefore, if a full workup has not identified the issue but symptoms persist, surgical exploration and revision may be necessary.

Pump related complications are less common. These can include a low volume pump [84], empty baclofen pump, failure of low battery alarm, rotating or "flipped" pump [76], stalled rotor or unknown causes [85]. These can be assessed by interrogating the pump including checking residual volume against calculated residual (less evidence is available for what might suggest a pump malfunction but ±15% may be a reason-able estimate for a functioning pump in an asymptomatic patient [86]), imaging, and surgical exploration and possible revision if symptoms persist. Temperature may also affect the flow rate of the pump.

Cavity related complications are the second most common cause of revisions and the most common cause for early readmission, more specifically wound and infection related episodes [87]. Protocol initiation has been shown to help decrease the rate of infection [88]. Subfascial placement in children and low weight individuals has been another method shown to decrease the rate of wound complications [72]. Early lumbar pseudomeningoceles occur most commonly in pediatric patients and can often be managed conservatively with bed rest and pressure dressings. Late presenta-tions should raise the suspicion of catheter migration [76]. Abdominal collections early may be related to seromas or hematomas, but an infection should be ruled out on clinical grounds with imaging and aspiration if needed. Late presentations may be a sign of catheter dislodgement or fracture causing leakage. Superficial and deep wound infections should be managed with appropriate antibiotic coverage and if pump system contamination is suspected or wound breakdown is evident then consideration for surgical revision is warranted.

4.6 Troubleshooting and caution

In regard to baclofen pump dosing, the provider should be aware of how to iden-tify and manage withdrawal, toxicity, and tolerance [42, 82]. Signs and symptoms of withdrawal and toxicity can overlap in the late stages to include nausea and vomit-ing, altered mental status or coma, tremor, seizures, respiratory failure, cardiac and autonomic dysfunction, while multi-organ failure has been reported with baclofen withdrawal [42, 89], and death. Unfortunately, many centers do not have established protocols for managing baclofen withdrawal [90].

Withdrawal; a decrease or—even more severe, a complete cessation of baclofen has resulted in significant morbidity and in mortality [91]. Causes can include failure to refill the pump, pump malfunction, catheter fracture/obstruction, arachnoid scarring, and at times is hard to definitively identify a cause. Early or milder symptoms can include pruritus, hyperthermia, hypertonia, and rhabdomyolysis. When suspicion is present that baclofen withdrawal has occurred/is occurring, rapid management is of the utmost importance. This includes supportive therapy as needed with close cardiorespiratory monitoring, beginning oral/enteral baclofen, the use of intravenous benzodiazepams as needed, and potentially intrathecal injection/infusion of baclofen while the pump is investigated for malfunction as above [82]. Symptoms and signs of baclofen withdrawal include early and late presentations, but the timing between the first appearance of symptoms which can occur within hours and life-threatening status can be 1 to 3 days.

Toxicity is more difficult to relate to any specific dose as this can vary from one individual to another and unlike oral baclofen, blood levels are a less accurate representation of the true CNS concentration. Causes can include pump malfunction, pump settings with recent adjustments being higher than tolerated, injecting into the access port and delivering a bolus dose. Signs and symptoms more suggestive of overdose include hypothermia, hypotonia, and hyporeflexia. Management includes supportive therapy with close cardiorespiratory monitoring as needed, discontinuation of baclofen until symptoms resolves (by stopping pump or aspirating reservoir to empty pump), consideration of lumbar puncture or CSF aspiration from access hub for CSF withdrawal to decrease the CSF concentration of the drug (20–30 mL), and intravenous benzodiazepams for any seizures.

Tolerance is even less defined, and is considered when higher doses are needed over time to achieve similar results, however, the main reason for such presentation should always be pump malfunction until proven otherwise through a stepwise approach. Once patency and appropriate function is confirmed, a lumbar puncture bolus trial can be attempted and in the absence of a good response this may be a consideration [89].

5. Spasticity: Neurosurgical management—Selective dorsal rhizotomy

5.1 History, mechanism, and indications

In order to understand the mechanism behind selective dorsal rhizotomy, a more detailed understanding of spasticity is needed. Charles Sherrington published his work in physiology through animal trials in 1898, whereby disconnecting the cortex from the spine at the level of the brainstem, led to "rigidity" in the limbs that was then relieved by sectioning of the innervating peripheral nerve [92]. Several years later, Liddell and Sherrington showed the importance of the stretch reflex [93]. There is a positive linear correlation between the speed of stretching the muscle and EMG activity found in the muscle, similar to what is appreciated in clinical practice, and therefore spasticity is considered a velocity-dependent phenomenon [94]. Although our understanding of spasticity drivers continues to evolve, the likely mechanism involves a loss of control of the spinal reflex where afferent neurons stimulate alpha motor neurons without the dampening effect of the spinal, suprasegmental, or supraspinal pathways due to some injury along these tracts (chief among them the reticulospinal tract) [95]. Taking advantage of this understanding of spasticity, many surgeons used neurotomy during the 1920 to 1970s to treat spasticity with good results, including cervical and lumbar procedures, most notable of whom was Otfrid Foerster [96]. However, the side effect profile at the time, including sensory and proprioception loss, bladder denervation, and atrophy as well as the introduction of other procedures and medications (e.g., Baclofen, Botulinum toxin, and Dantrolene) may have limited its further spread and utilization by the end of the twentieth century. A more detailed account of the evolution of selective dorsal rhizotomy (SDR) is presented elsewhere [97, 98].

As the understanding and utilization of neuromonitoring and stimulation continued to advance and become incorporated into spasticity surgery [99–101], Warwick Peacock described a multi-level approach to selectively section the exiting dorsal nerve roots thereby minimizing the complications of prior techniques [102]. He was recruited from Cape Town to University of California, Los Angeles and introduced his technique to centers across the United States [97]. The two major contributions thereafter came from T.S. Park who performed the procedure similar to its original description at the level of the conus but used EMG guided sectioning of the dorsal nerve roots [103], and from Marc Sindou from Lyon, France who performed a key-hole interlaminar dorsal rhizotomy to minimize disruption of the posterior elements of the spinal column [104]. A review of these and other techniques are presented elsewhere [105].

Indications to perform SDR are not standardized [106], but candidates are generally divided into two main groups. The first are individuals with spastic diplegia that are ambulatory. The objective here is to improve functional outcomes and alleviate lower limb tone that may be limiting certain activities and to assist with mobility. Often done before 12 years of age, there is no definitive answer regarding optimal timing. The youngest age for consideration of the procedure is thought to be 2–3 years of age and many believe 4–6 years is ideal as children are motivated and have not yet started school and earlier intervention may help prevent musculoskeletal changes that occur with spasticity over time, but it is also performed in older children and adults with good results [107, 108]. One study with a smaller sample size did raise the concern for decline in function after SDR in individuals with spastic diplegia who had surgery between 10 and 20 years of age [109], but this has not been reported by others.

To obtain the best outcome in these individuals, appropriate selection is important. Firstly, individuals should be assessed by a multidisciplinary team to confirm the diagnosis and that spasticity of the lower extremities is the major component of their hypertonia as other types of hypertonia will not respond to the procedure and those with a prominent dystonia component may worsen after SDR. Secondly, the ability from the patient and commitment from the family to be involved in postoperative rehabilitation as the decrease in tone will often lead to a decline in function before gains are achieved with training. Thirdly, that the child is not using their hypertonia to compensate for any muscle weakness thereby having a positive effect on function which would worsen if the tone were decreased and conversely that contractures or a limited range of motion is present to prevent optimal physiotherapy that may benefit from orthopedic intervention prior to SDR. The second group are non-ambulatory individuals (GMFCS 4 and 5), who more often have spastic tetraplegia or quadriplegia. In these individuals, SDR may play a role in facilitating care for bathing, transfers, and seating as severe spasticity and clonus can make these daily tasks challenging, and improving their quality of life. This may be an option for individuals who are not candidates for baclofen pumps and whose main concerns are the spasticity of the lower more so than the upper limbs.

5.2 Evidence and long-term outcomes

A meta-analysis of three randomized control trials (RCT) that included individuals with GMFCS 1 to 4, comparing SDR and physiotherapy with physiotherapy alone, showed that SDR and physiotherapy significantly reduce tone based on the Ashworth score and improve GMFM scores at 9–12 months compared to physiotherapy alone, providing class 1 evidence for its application in spasticity [110]. A more recent RCT also found that SDR followed by physiotherapy had better function at 1 year than physiotherapy alone in ambulatory children [111]. An observational study in the United Kingdom over a 2 year period including children GMFCS 2 and 3 found a significant improvement in GMFM-66 scores and quality of life scores in those undergoing SDR, which helped pass a national policy to fund this procedure in eligible children [112]. Longer term studies at 5 years [113], 10 years [114], 15 years [115], and even 20 years [108] reported sustained benefit in regard to decreased tone and functional scores. However, the evidence for its effect on long-term functional outcome remains less conclusive based on current publishes studies. One long term study found that 5–10 years after SDR, some individuals had more than expected improvement in function, and that no individual had any worse than expected outcomes. A matched cohort survey that examined individuals who underwent SDR and those who did not, found similar improvement in gait at 10 to 18 years in both groups but significantly less interventions in the SDR group [116]. This study was limited by a smaller sample size of 35 individuals. A similar study assessed 88 individuals with CP and was a case-control study for SDR and non-SDR groups and found that those who underwent SDR as children had a positive functional impact compared to their matched control group [117]. A systemic review concluded that as of 2018, no high quality studies were available to make definitive statements about long term benefits of the procedure, but shorter term evidence of its benefit are more robust [118]. This is likely related to variability across studies in regard to selection criteria, GMFCS levels included, surgical technique and outcome measures. In addition to its effects on the lower limbs, suprasegmental effects to decrease tone in the upper extremities has also been noted by several groups over the years [119].

The effect of SDR on the rate of orthopedic surgeries for spasticity is variable as some groups may require less lifetime interventions while others have similar rates to their non-SDR cohorts and this is likely related to age at surgery and ambulatory status. Some evidence suggests that younger age for SDR (2–4 years) may decrease the need for orthopedic surgeries [108]. Others found similar findings in those aged 4–5 year compared to their cohorts who did not have an SDR [116], and potentially in children younger than 10 years [115]. Further high quality studies are needed, but there may be a benefit in decreasing the number of orthopedic interventions needed for children with a good functional status and ambulation if SDR is done early.

Whether SDR accelerates scoliosis or increases the need for surgical intervention is also less clear and likely similarly related to natural history of individuals with CP, age at surgery, functional status, and preoperative curve [120]. Some evidence suggests that SDR does not worsen the natural history [121], while others concluded that multi-level approaches may increase the risk while single levels approaches may be protective [108]. A retrospective study comparing single and multi-level approaches found only a difference in length of stay favoring the single level approach [122]. Some evidence also shows that SDR helps improve bladder function in regard to urgency, frequency, and incontinence [123].

Neurosurgical Management of Spasticity
DOI: http://dx.doi.org/10.5772/intechopen.1010933

5.3 Surgical techniques, postoperative pain control, and complications

The surgical techniques for SDR have been reported elsewhere, and exposure of the target nerves can be through a single (**Figures 8–10**) or multiple level approach through a laminectomy, laminoplasty, or keyhole approach [105, 124, 125]. Here we will discuss the evidence and reports of variations in the surgical techniques.

The basis of the surgical approach for SDR is to selectively section enough rootlets at any given level to achieve a decrease in the targeted muscle tone—this involves sectioning *enough* rootlets at each level to achieve an effective long-term response and to avoid sectioning *too many* rootlets to cause more profound hypotonia and loss of sensation/proprioception. The best percentage to cut is unknown but often guided by ambulatory status (more conservative) and non-ambulatory status (more aggressive) as these two groups have different goals from SDR. Some advocate a standard sectioning of ~2/3rd of each sensory nerve [124], but reports vary widely (from 0% to 90%) based on EMG response [121, 126], while some have modified their technique over time and varies based on level [127, 128]. A comparative study between sectioning 50% of target nerve roots versus less than 50% showed a potential benefit in gait secondary to improved ankle power in the more conservative approach [129]. However, no definitive data exists to know the optimal number of rootlets to section and is likely patient and nerve root per patient specific and further data is needed to clarify this further.

SDR includes sectioning from L2 to S1 and many recommend including L1 and S2 roots as well. Including L1 in the rhizotomy is recommended as this may be a contributor to hip flexor spasticity [124], although some have found no significant difference in sectioning versus preservation [130]. Not including S2 in SDR has been showed to sometimes result in persistence of increased ankle tone in some individuals

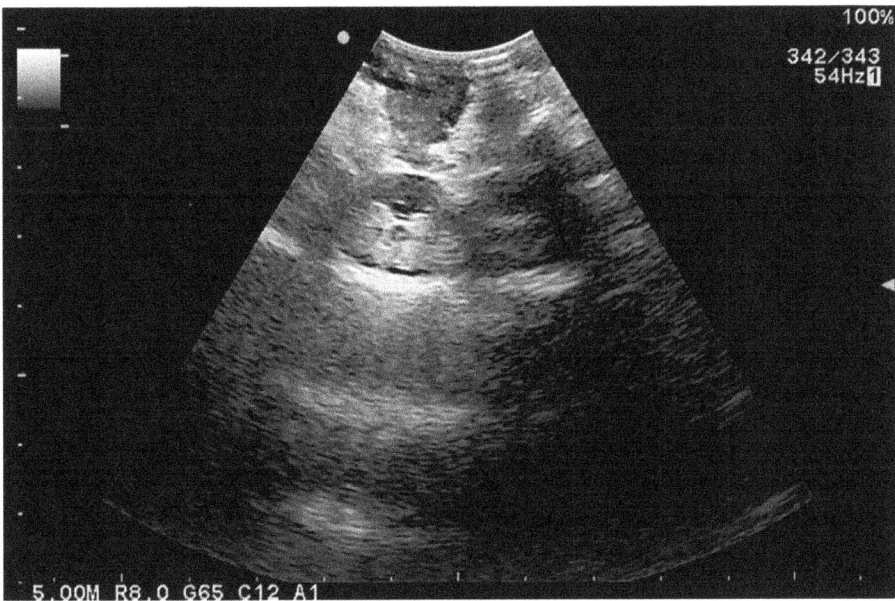

Figure 8.
Epidural ultrasound after opening the interlaminar space to confirm transitional level of the conus and cauda equina.

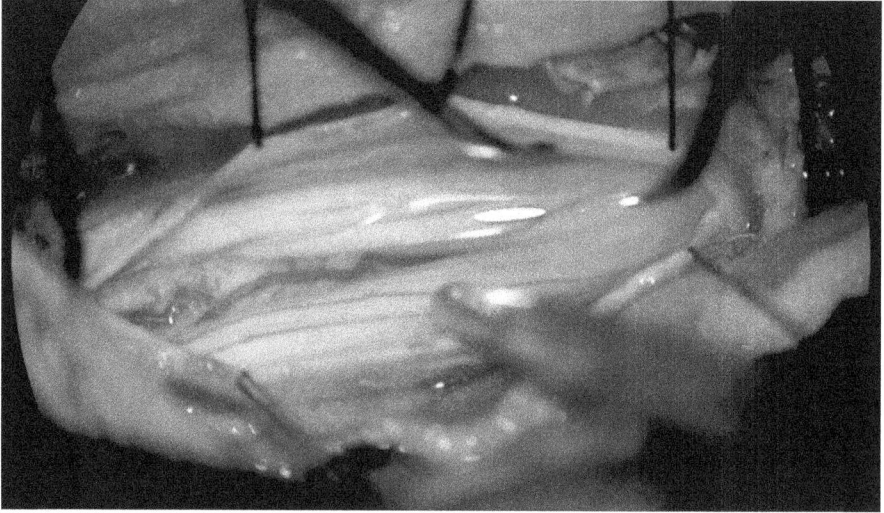

Figure 9.
Single level laminectomy at the level of the transition and the dura is open to expose the intradural components. Seen on the left-hand side is the conus and on the right-hand side is the cauda equina.

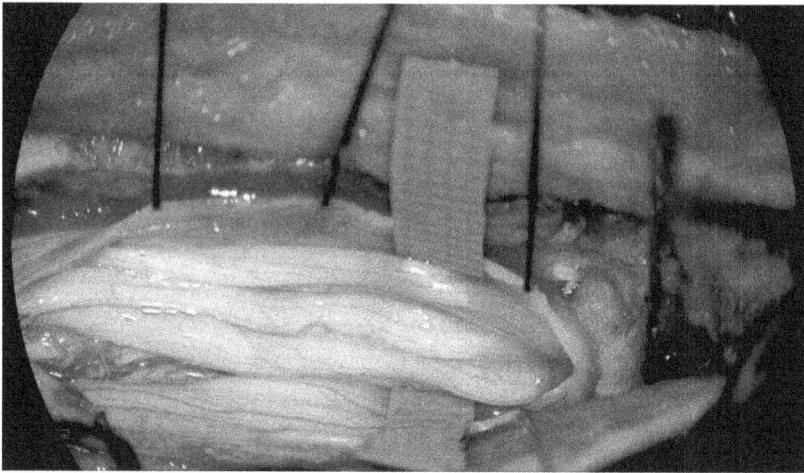

Figure 10.
Silastic sheet used to isolate the right dorsal nerve roots. Smaller midline lower sacral nerve roots are spared and note included in the rhizotomy.

postoperatively and therefore is recommended to be included in the SDR with similar precautions to ensure no lower sacral nerves are included [113, 130].

Intraoperative neuromonitoring (IONM) is often used during SDR. A rhizotomy probe (right angle stimulator with a cathode and anode) can be used to localize the nerve root based on EMG response, followed by dividing the nerve root into rootlets and stimulating each rootlet at 50 Hz and grading the response from 0 to 4 based on prior descriptions by Phillips and Park (**Figures 11** and **12**) [131]. This should be performed at a center where the neurosurgeon and neuromonitoring team are familiar with the procedure, stimulation parameters and interpretation of the responses, taking into account the patient specific preoperative assessment. Many consider grades 3 and 4 (more severe) to be included in the rhizotomy while 0–2 (normal to moderate) may be preserved, the percentage of course differing across centers based on the above discussion. However, IONM is also debated to its usefulness by some [132, 133], but there exists several publication in strong support of its use [104, 125, 134, 135].

Postoperative pain control is important as patients can experience a burning dysesthesia in the lower extremities after the procedure. A recent systematic review on various options including pumps and epidural analgesia is reported [136], and multi-modal analgesia including epidural administration of non-opioid drugs likely has the best response and lower side effect profile. SDR has been shown to be a safe procedure, but complications from SDR are not uncommonly reported across studies although these are generally mild. Two systemic reviews examined

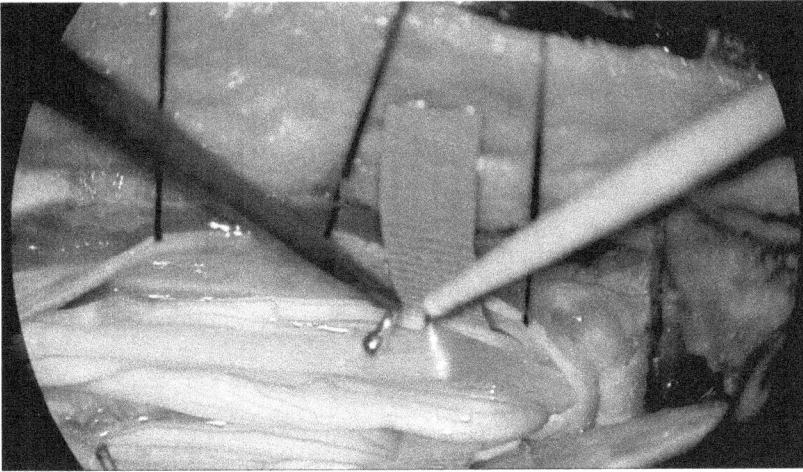

Figure 11.
Stimulation of the nerve root to identify the level and confirm that a dorsal nerve root is selected and not a ventral nerve root.

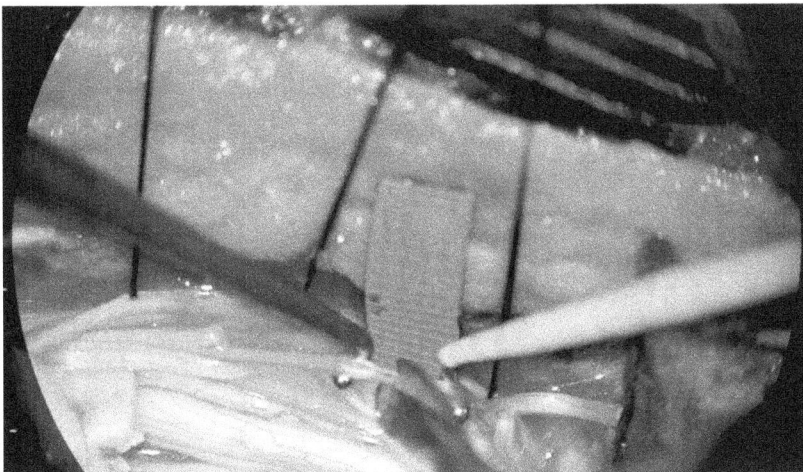

Figure 12.
After separating the nerve root into rootlets and stimulating the rootlet to identify abnormal from a normal response, the rootlet is then cut.

published reports and complications can include constipation, bladder dysfunction, and sensory changes in less than 10–15% [118, 137].

6. Other neurosurgical options for spasticity

Several case series have investigated the cerebellar dentate nuclei as a target for deep brain stimulation in individuals with CP and movement disorders. The cerebellums' role in movement and its cortical and subcortical connections through the superior cerebellar peduncle form the basis of this targeting. Several studies have shown a positive effect in lowering muscle tone, improvement in dystonia, and quality of life for individuals with CP [138–142]. However, further evidence is needed prior to including this as an option in the neurosurgeon's armamentarium for managing spasticity.

7. Conclusions

Spasticity is the most common movement disorder present in individuals with CP and can have a negative impact on function and quality of life. Two neurosurgical procedures are available to help manage spasticity, Baclofen pumps which are a reversible intervention and selective dorsal rhizotomy which is a non-reversible intervention. Baclofen pumps for appropriately selected candidates can make a meaningful impact on spasticity control and quality of life, especially for spasticity involving all four limbs, but requires close monitoring and follow up. SDR is proven to be effective in spasticity relief of the lower extremities and improved function and quality of life with potential suprasegmental effects in the upper extremities. Its effect on the rate of orthopedic surgeries, scoliosis surgery, and bladder function varies based on available reports and further high-quality research is needed. Referral to a specialized center for individuals with CP for multidisciplinary assessment can help provide patients and their families with available options to help achieve better outcomes.

Conflict of interest

The author declares no conflict of interest.

Neurosurgical Management of Spasticity
DOI: http://dx.doi.org/10.5772/intechopen.1010933

Author details

Ziyad Makoshi[1,2]

1 Neuroscience Department, El Paso Children's Hospital, El Paso, Texas, USA

2 Paul L. Foster School of Medicine, Texas Tech University Health Sciences Center El Paso, El Paso, Texas, USA

*Address all correspondence to: ziyad.makoshi@elpasochildrens.org

IntechOpen

References

[1] Sanger TD et al. Classification and definition of disorders causing hypertonia in childhood. Pediatrics. 2003;**111**(1):e89-e97

[2] Ganguly J et al. Muscle tone physiology and abnormalities. Toxins. 2021;**13**(4):282

[3] Hart AR et al. Neonatal hypertonia— A diagnostic challenge. Developmental Medicine and Child Neurology. 2015;**57**(7):600-610

[4] Morris C. Definition and classification of cerebral palsy: A historical perspective. Developmental Medicine and Child Neurology. Supplement. 2007;**109**:3-7

[5] Raju TN. Historical perspectives on the etiology of cerebral palsy. Clinics in Perinatology. 2006;**33**(2):233-250

[6] Wilkins RH, Brody IA. Little's disease. Archives of Neurology. 1969;**20**(2):217-224

[7] Osler W. Cerebral Palsies of Children. United Kingdom: Mac Keith Press; 1889

[8] Accardo PJ. Freud on diplegia. Commentary and translation. American Journal of Diseases of Children. 1982;**136**(5):452-456

[9] Wolf J. Historical perspective of cerebral palsy. In: The Results of Treatment in Cerebral Palsy. Springfield, IL: Charles C Thomas; 1969

[10] Bax MC. Terminology and classification of cerebral palsy. Developmental Medicine and Child Neurology. 1964;**6**:295-297

[11] Mutch L et al. Cerebral palsy epidemiology: Where are we now and where are we going? Developmental Medicine and Child Neurology. 1992;**34**(6):547-551

[12] Surveillance of Cerebral Palsy in Europe. Surveillance of cerebral palsy in Europe: A collaboration of cerebral palsy surveys and registers. Surveillance of Cerebral Palsy in Europe (SCPE). Developmental Medicine and Child Neurology. 2000;**42**(12):816-824

[13] Bax M et al. Proposed definition and classification of cerebral palsy, April 2005. Developmental Medicine and Child Neurology. 2005;**47**(8):571-576

[14] Donald KA et al. Pediatric cerebral palsy in Africa: A systematic review. Seminars in Pediatric Neurology. 2014;**21**(1):30-35

[15] Barron-Garza F et al. Incidence of cerebral palsy, risk factors, and neuroimaging in Northeast Mexico. Pediatric Neurology. 2023;**143**:50-58

[16] Olusanya BO et al. Global prevalence of developmental disabilities in children and adolescents: A systematic umbrella review. Frontiers in Public Health. 2023;**11**:1122009

[17] Minear WL. A classification of cerebral palsy. Pediatrics. 1956;**18**(5):841-852

[18] Pandyan AD et al. Spasticity: Clinical perceptions, neurological realities and meaningful measurement. Disability and Rehabilitation. 2005;**27**(1-2):2-6

[19] Johnson A. Prevalence and characteristics of children with cerebral palsy in Europe. Developmental Medicine and Child Neurology. 2002;**44**(9):633-640

[20] Reid SM, Carlin JB, Reddihough DS. Classification of topographical pattern

of spasticity in cerebral palsy: A registry perspective. Research in Developmental Disabilities. 2011;**32**(6):2909-2915

[21] Reid SM, Carlin JB, Reddihough DS. Distribution of motor types in cerebral palsy: How do registry data compare? Developmental Medicine and Child Neurology. 2011;**53**(3):233-238

[22] Hagglund G, Wagner P. Development of spasticity with age in a total population of children with cerebral palsy. BMC Musculoskeletal Disorders. 2008;**9**:150

[23] Linden O et al. The development of spasticity with age in 4,162 children with cerebral palsy: A register-based prospective cohort study. Acta Orthopaedica. 2019;**90**(3):286-291

[24] Pierce SR, Prosser LA, Lauer RT. Relationship between age and spasticity in children with diplegic cerebral palsy. Archives of Physical Medicine and Rehabilitation. 2010;**91**(3):448-451

[25] Beckung E et al. The natural history of gross motor development in children with cerebral palsy aged 1 to 15 years. Developmental Medicine and Child Neurology. 2007;**49**(10):751-756

[26] Hanna SE et al. Stability and decline in gross motor function among children and youth with cerebral palsy aged 2 to 21 years. Developmental Medicine and Child Neurology. 2009;**51**(4):295-302

[27] Rosenbaum PL et al. Prognosis for gross motor function in cerebral palsy: Creation of motor development curves. JAMA. 2002;**288**(11):1357-1363

[28] Ashworth B. Preliminary trial of carisoprodol in multiple sclerosis. Practitioner. 1964;**192**:540-542

[29] Bohannon RW, Smith MB. Interrater reliability of a modified Ashworth scale

of muscle spasticity. Physical Therapy. 1987;**67**(2):206-207

[30] Russell DJ et al. The gross motor function measure: A means to evaluate the effects of physical therapy. Developmental Medicine and Child Neurology. 1989;**31**(3):341-352

[31] Russell DJ, Wright M, Rosenbaum PL, Avery LM. Gross Motor Function Measure (GMFM-66 & GMFM-88) User's Manual, 3rd Edition. United Kingdom: John Wiley and Sons; Sep 2021. p. 336

[32] Palisano R et al. Development and reliability of a system to classify gross motor function in children with cerebral palsy. Developmental Medicine and Child Neurology. 1997;**39**(4):214-223

[33] Nicoll RA. My close encounter with GABA(B) receptors. Biochemical Pharmacology. 2004;**68**(8):1667-1674

[34] Bormann J. The 'ABC' of GABA receptors. Trends in Pharmacological Sciences. 2000;**21**(1):16-19

[35] Colombo G. GABAB Receptor. Vol. 29. Switzerland: Springer; 2016

[36] Spiering MJ. The discovery of GABA in the brain. The Journal of Biological Chemistry. 2018;**293**(49):19159-19160

[37] Salim SA et al. Baclofen-induced neurotoxicity in patients with compromised renal function: Review. International Journal of Clinical Pharmacology and Therapeutics. 2018;**56**(10):467-475

[38] Benarroch EE. GABAB receptors: Structure, functions, and clinical implications. Neurology. 2012;**78**(8):578-584

[39] Zuzan O, Leuwer M. 12 Neuromuscular blocking agents and skeletal muscle relaxants. In: Aronson

J editor. Side Effects of Drugs Annual. Vol. 29. The Netherlands: Elsevier; 2007. pp. 155-159

[40] Abdel-Magid AF. Therapeutic advantage of the positive allosteric modulators of the GABA-B receptor. ACS Medicinal Chemistry Letters. 2017;**8**(5):474-475

[41] Albright AL. Neurosurgical treatment of spasticity: Selective posterior rhizotomy and intrathecal baclofen. Stereotactic and Functional Neurosurgery. 1992;**58**(1-4):3-13

[42] Romito JW et al. Baclofen therapeutics, toxicity, and withdrawal: A narrative review. SAGE Open Medicine. 2021;**9**:20503121211022197

[43] Saulino M et al. Best practices for intrathecal baclofen therapy: Patient selection. Neuromodulation. 2016;**19**(6):607-615

[44] Boster AL et al. Best practices for intrathecal baclofen therapy: Screening test. Neuromodulation. 2016;**19**(6):616-622

[45] Berweck S et al. Use of intrathecal baclofen in children and adolescents: Interdisciplinary consensus table 2013. Neuropediatrics. 2014;**45**(5):294-308

[46] Albright AL, Cervi A, Singletary J. Intrathecal baclofen for spasticity in cerebral palsy. JAMA. 1991;**265**(11): 1418-1422

[47] Dralle D et al. Intrathecal baclofen for spasticity. Lancet. 1985;**2**(8462):1003

[48] Dralle D, Neuhauser G, Tonn JC. Intrathecal baclofen for cerebral spasticity. Lancet. 1989;**2**(8668):916

[49] Hasnat MJ, Rice JE. Intrathecal baclofen for treating spasticity in children with cerebral palsy. Cochrane Database of Systematic Reviews. 2015;**11**:CD004552

[50] Albright AL et al. Continuous intrathecal baclofen infusion for spasticity of cerebral origin. JAMA. 1993;**270**(20):2475-2477

[51] Albright AL et al. Effects of continuous intrathecal baclofen infusion and selective posterior rhizotomy on upper extremity spasticity. Pediatric Neurosurgery. 1995;**23**(2):82-85

[52] Albright AL. Baclofen in the treatment of cerebral palsy. Journal of Child Neurology. 1996;**11**(2):77-83

[53] Kraus T et al. Long-term therapy with intrathecal baclofen improves quality of life in children with severe spastic cerebral palsy. European Journal of Paediatric Neurology. 2017;**21**(3):565-569

[54] Krach LE, Nettleton A, Klempka B. Satisfaction of individuals treated long-term with continuous infusion of intrathecal baclofen by implanted programmable pump. Pediatric Rehabilitation. 2006;**9**(3):210-218

[55] Campbell WM et al. Long-term safety and efficacy of continuous intrathecal baclofen. Developmental Medicine and Child Neurology. 2002;**44**(10):660-665

[56] Masrour M et al. Intrathecal baclofen efficacy for managing motor function and spasticity severity in patients with cerebral palsy: A systematic review and meta-analysis. BMC Neurology. 2024;**24**(1):143

[57] Dario A, Tomei G. A benefit-risk assessment of baclofen in severe spinal spasticity. Drug Safety. 2004;**27**(11):799-818

[58] Medical Advisory S. Intrathecal baclofen pump for spasticity: An evidence-based analysis. Ontario Health Technology Assessment Series. 2005;**5**(7):1-93

[59] Lee S et al. Effect of intrathecal baclofen pump on scoliosis in children with cerebral palsy: A meta-analysis. Annals of Rehabilitation Medicine. 2023;**47**(1):11-18

[60] Gerszten PC, Albright AL, Johnstone GF. Intrathecal baclofen infusion and subsequent orthopedic surgery in patients with spastic cerebral palsy. Journal of Neurosurgery. 1998;**88**(6):1009-1013

[61] Gooch JL, McFadden M, Oberg W. Orthopedic surgery in children with intrathecal baclofen pumps. Journal of Pediatric Rehabilitation Medicine. 2013;**6**(4):233-238

[62] Asma A et al. Does intrathecal baclofen therapy decrease the progression of hip displacement in young patients with cerebral palsy? Developmental Medicine and Child Neurology. 2023;**65**(8):1112-1117

[63] Atkinson C, Rawicki B, Low N. The role of tissue expansion before baclofen pump insertion in the pediatric population. Annals of Plastic Surgery. 2024;**93**(5):611-616

[64] Albright AL, Turner M, Pattisapu JV. Best-practice surgical techniques for intrathecal baclofen therapy. Journal of Neurosurgery. 2006;**104**(4 Suppl):233-239

[65] Haranhalli N et al. Intrathecal baclofen therapy: Complication avoidance and management. Child's Nervous System. 2011;**27**(3):421-427

[66] Klimo P Jr et al. Pediatric hydrocephalus: Systematic literature review and evidence-based guidelines. Part 6: Preoperative antibiotics for shunt surgery in children with hydrocephalus: A systematic review and meta-analysis. Journal of Neurosurgery. Pediatrics. 2014;**14** (Suppl. 1):44-52

[67] Sarmey N et al. Evidence-based interventions to reduce shunt infections: A systematic review. Child's Nervous System. 2015;**31**(4):541-549

[68] Follett KA et al. Prevention of intrathecal drug delivery catheter-related complications. Neuromodulation. 2003;**6**(1):32-41

[69] Borowski A et al. Baclofen pump implantation and spinal fusion in children: Techniques and complications. Spine (Phila Pa 1976). 2008;**33**(18):1995-2000

[70] Liu JK, Walker ML. Posterior cervical approach for intrathecal baclofen pump insertion in children with previous spinal fusions. Technical note. Journal of Neurosurgery. 2005;**102**(1 Suppl):119-122

[71] Turner M, Nguyen HS, Cohen-Gadol AA. Intraventricular baclofen as an alternative to intrathecal baclofen for intractable spasticity or dystonia: Outcomes and technical considerations. Journal of Neurosurgery. Pediatrics. 2012;**10**(4):315-319

[72] Kopell BH et al. Subfascial implantation of intrathecal baclofen pumps in children: Technical note. Neurosurgery. 2001;**49**(3):753-756; discussion 756-7

[73] Nuru M et al. Infectious complications and operative management of intrathecal baclofen pumps in the pediatric population: A systematic review and meta-analysis of 20 years of pooled experience. World Neurosurgery. 2022;**163**:e59-e72

[74] Ricciardelli A et al. Peritoneal baclofen pump migration: A rare complication of subfascial placement. Illustrative cases. Journal of Neurosurgery: Case Lessons. 2024;**8**(10):CASE24290

[75] Bogue JT et al. Submuscular placement of baclofen infusion pumps: Case series and technique. Annals of Plastic Surgery. 2020;**85** (Suppl. 1):S8-S11

[76] Vender JR et al. Identification and management of intrathecal baclofen pump complications: A comparison of pediatric and adult patients. Journal of Neurosurgery. 2006;**104**(Suppl. 1):9-15

[77] Cobourn KD et al. Use of intraoperative topical antibiotics to reduce intrathecal baclofen pump surgical site infections: A single institution's experience over 24 years. Journal of Neurosurgery. Pediatrics. 2023;**32**(1):69-74

[78] Spader HS et al. Risk factors for baclofen pump infection in children: A multivariate analysis. Journal of Neurosurgery. Pediatrics. 2016;**17**(6):756-762

[79] Awaad Y et al. Complications of intrathecal baclofen pump: Prevention and cure. ISRN Neurology. 2012;**2012**:575168

[80] Ammar A et al. Intrathecal baclofen therapy—How we do it. Journal of Neurosurgery. Pediatrics. 2012;**10**(5):439-444

[81] Miracle AC et al. Imaging evaluation of intrathecal baclofen pump-catheter systems. AJNR. American Journal of Neuroradiology. 2011;**32**(7):1158-1164

[82] Saulino M et al. Best practices for intrathecal baclofen therapy: Troubleshooting. Neuromodulation. 2016;**19**(6):632-641

[83] Dawes WJ, Drake JM, Fehlings D. Microfracture of a baclofen pump catheter with intermittent under- and overdose. Pediatric Neurosurgery. 2003;**39**(3):144-148

[84] Rigoli G, Terrini G, Cordioli Z. Intrathecal baclofen withdrawal syndrome caused by low residual volume in the pump reservoir: A report of 2 cases. Archives of Physical Medicine and Rehabilitation. 2004;**85**(12):2064-2066

[85] Borowski A et al. Complications of intrathecal baclofen pump therapy in pediatric patients. Journal of Pediatric Orthopedics. 2010;**30**(1):76-81

[86] Wesemann K et al. Clinical accuracy and safety using the SynchroMed II intrathecal drug infusion pump. Regional Anesthesia and Pain Medicine. 2014;**39**(4):341-346

[87] Lam SK et al. Readmission and complications within 30 days after intrathecal baclofen pump placement. Developmental Medicine and Child Neurology. 2018;**60**(10):1038-1044

[88] Desai VR et al. A standardized protocol to reduce pediatric baclofen pump infections: A quality improvement initiative. Journal of Neurosurgery. Pediatrics. 2018;**21**(4):395-400

[89] Kaye AD et al. Efficacy, indications, and safety of intrathecal baclofen pump: A narrative review. Current Pain and Headache Reports. 2025;**29**(1):9

[90] Schmitz NS et al. Characterizing baclofen withdrawal: A national survey of physician experience. Pediatric Neurology. 2021;**122**:106-109

[91] Mohammed I, Hussain A. Intrathecal baclofen withdrawal syndrome- a life-threatening complication of baclofen pump: A case report. BMC Clinical Pharmacology. 2004;**4**:6

[92] Sherrington CS. Decerebrate rigidity, and reflex coordination of movements. The Journal of Physiology. 1898;**22**(4):319-332

[93] Rushworth G. Some studies on the pathophysiology of spasticity. Spinal Cord. 1966;**4**(3):130-141

[94] Trompetto C et al. Pathophysiology of spasticity: Implications for neurorehabilitation. BioMed Research International. 2014;**2014**:354906

[95] Mukherjee A, Chakravarty A. Spasticity mechanisms—For the clinician. Frontiers in Neurology. 2010;**1**:149

[96] Foerster. Resection of the posterior spinal nerve-roots in the treatment of gastric crises and spastic paralysis. Proceedings of the Royal Society of Medicine. 1911;**4**(Surg Sect):254

[97] Enslin JMN, Langerak NG, Fieggen AG. The evolution of selective dorsal rhizotomy for the management of spasticity. Neurotherapeutics. 2019;**16**(1):3-8

[98] Cespedes J et al. History and evolution of surgical treatment for spasticity: A journey from neurotomy to selective dorsal rhizotomy. Neurosurgical Focus. 2024;**56**(6):E2

[99] Fasano VA et al. Surgical treatment of spasticity in cerebral palsy. Child's Brain. 1978;**4**(5):289-305

[100] Fasano VA et al. Electrophysiological assessment of spinal circuits in spasticity by direct dorsal root stimulation. Neurosurgery. 1979;**4**(2):146-151

[101] Gros C et al. Selective posterior radicotomy in the neurosurgical treatment of pyramidal hypertension. Neurochirurgie. 1967;**13**(4):505-518

[102] Peacock WJ, Arens LJ. Selective posterior rhizotomy for the relief of spasticity in cerebral palsy. South African Medical Journal. 1982;**62**(4):119-124

[103] Park TS et al. Selective lumbosacral dorsal rhizotomy immediately caudal to the conus medullaris for cerebral palsy spasticity. Neurosurgery. 1993;**33**(5):929-933; discussion 933-4

[104] Georgoulis G, Brînzeu A, Sindou M. Dorsal rhizotomy for children with spastic diplegia of cerebral palsy origin: Usefulness of intraoperative monitoring. Journal of Neurosurgery. Pediatrics. 2018;**22**(1):89-101

[105] Warsi NM et al. Selective dorsal rhizotomy: An illustrated review of operative techniques. Journal of Neurosurgery. Pediatrics. 2020:**25**(5):540-547

[106] Grunt S et al. Selection criteria for selective dorsal rhizotomy in children with spastic cerebral palsy: A systematic review of the literature. Developmental Medicine and Child Neurology. 2014;**56**(4):302-312

[107] Makoshi Z et al. A mixed methods study of practice variation in selective dorsal rhizotomy: A study by the cerebral palsy research network. Pediatric Neurology. 2023;**149**:159-166

[108] Park TS et al. Functional outcome of adulthood selective dorsal rhizotomy for spastic diplegia. Cureus. 2019;**11**(7):e5184

[109] MacWilliams BA et al. Functional decline in children undergoing selective dorsal rhizotomy after age 10. Developmental Medicine and Child Neurology. 2011;**53**(8):717-723

[110] McLaughlin J et al. Selective dorsal rhizotomy: Meta-analysis of

three randomized controlled trials. Developmental Medicine and Child Neurology. 2002;**44**(1):17-25

[111] Abd-Elmonem AM et al. Effect of physical training on motor function of ambulant children with diplegia after selective dorsal rhizotomy: A randomized controlled study. NeuroRehabilitation. 2023;**53**(4):547-556

[112] Summers J et al. Selective dorsal rhizotomy in ambulant children with cerebral palsy: An observational cohort study. The Lancet Child & Adolescent Health. 2019;**3**(7):455-462

[113] Nordmark E et al. Long-term outcomes five years after selective dorsal rhizotomy. BMC Pediatrics. 2008;**8**:54

[114] Ailon T et al. Long-term outcome after selective dorsal rhizotomy in children with spastic cerebral palsy. Child's Nervous System. 2015;**31**(3):415-423

[115] Dudley RW et al. Long-term functional benefits of selective dorsal rhizotomy for spastic cerebral palsy. Journal of Neurosurgery. Pediatrics. 2013;**12**(2):142-150

[116] Munger ME et al. Long-term outcomes after selective dorsal rhizotomy: A retrospective matched cohort study. Developmental Medicine and Child Neurology. 2017;**59**(11):1196-1203

[117] Daunter AK, Kratz AL, Hurvitz EA. Long-term impact of childhood selective dorsal rhizotomy on pain, fatigue, and function: A case-control study. Developmental Medicine and Child Neurology. 2017;**59**(10):1089-1095

[118] Tedroff K, Hagglund G, Miller F. Long-term effects of selective dorsal rhizotomy in children with cerebral palsy: A systematic review. Developmental Medicine and Child Neurology. 2020;**62**(5):554-562

[119] Merckx L et al. Upper-extremity spasticity and functionality after selective dorsal rhizotomy for cerebral palsy: A systematic review. Journal of Neurosurgery. Pediatrics. 2023;**32**(6):673-685

[120] Ravindra VM et al. Risk factors for progressive neuromuscular scoliosis requiring posterior spinal fusion after selective dorsal rhizotomy. Journal of Neurosurgery. Pediatrics. 2017;**20**(5):456-463

[121] Miller SD et al. The effect of selective dorsal rhizotomy on scoliosis in children with cerebral palsy: A long-term follow-up study. Journal of Pediatric Orthopedics. 2025;**45**(3):158-163

[122] Ou C et al. Selective dorsal rhizotomy in children: Comparison of outcomes after single-level versus multi-level laminectomy technique. Canadian Journal of Neuroscience Nursing. 2010;**32**(3):17-24

[123] Chiu PK et al. Does selective dorsal rhizotomy improve bladder function in children with cerebral palsy? International Urology and Nephrology. 2014;**46**(10):1929-1933

[124] Park TS, Johnston JM. Surgical techniques of selective dorsal rhizotomy for spastic cerebral palsy. Technical note. Neurosurgical Focus. 2006;**21**(2):e7

[125] Makoshi Z et al. Postoperative outcomes and stimulation responses for sectioned nerve roots during selective dorsal rhizotomy in cerebral palsy. Acta Neurochirurgica. 2024;**166**(1):308

[126] Trost JP et al. Comprehensive short-term outcome assessment of selective dorsal rhizotomy. Developmental

Medicine and Child Neurology.
2008;**50**(10):765-771

[127] Kim HS, Steinbok P, Wickenheiser D.
Predictors of poor outcome after selective
dorsal rhizotomy in treatment of spastic
cerebral palsy. Child's Nervous System.
2006;**22**(1):60-66

[128] Steinbok P et al. Spinal deformities
after selective dorsal rhizotomy for
spastic cerebral palsy. Journal of
Neurosurgery. 2005;**102**
(Suppl. 4):363-373

[129] Mantese B et al. Selective dorsal
rhizotomy: Analysis of two rootlet
sectioning techniques. Child's Nervous
System. 2024;**40**(4):1147-1157

[130] Kim DS et al. Selective posterior
rhizotomy for lower extremity spasticity:
How much and which of the posterior
rootlets should be cut? Surgical
Neurology. 2002;**57**(2):87-93

[131] Phillips LH, Park TS.
Electrophysiologic mapping of the
segmental anatomy of the muscles of
the lower extremity. Muscle & Nerve.
1991;**14**(12):1213-1218

[132] Steinbok P et al. Electrophysiologically guided versus non-
electrophysiologically guided selective
dorsal rhizotomy for spastic cerebral
palsy: A comparison of outcomes. Child's
Nervous System. 2009;**25**(9):1091-1096

[133] Warf BC, Nelson KR. The
electromyographic responses to dorsal
rootlet stimulation during partial dorsal
rhizotomy are inconsistent. Pediatric
Neurosurgery. 1996;**25**(1):13-19

[134] Joud A et al. Dorsal rhizotomy in
cerebral palsy: How root sectioning
is influenced by intraoperative
neuromonitoring? Neurochirurgie.
2022;**68**(5):e16-e21

[135] Sindou M, Joud A, Georgoulis G.
Usefulness of external anal sphincter
EMG recording for intraoperative
neuromonitoring of the sacral
roots-a prospective study in dorsal
rhizotomy. Acta Neurochirurgica.
2021;**163**(2):479-487

[136] Lu VM, Vazquez S, Niazi TN.
Postoperative pain management
strategies following selective dorsal
rhizotomy in pediatric cerebral palsy
patients: A systematic review of
published regimens. Child's Nervous
System. 2024;**40**(12):4095-4105

[137] Mishra D et al. A systematic
review of complications following
selective dorsal rhizotomy in
cerebral palsy. Neurochirurgie.
2023;**69**(3):101425

[138] Cajigas I et al. Cerebellar deep
brain stimulation for the treatment
of movement disorders in cerebral
palsy. Journal of Neurosurgery.
2023;**139**(3):605-614

[139] Davis R. Cerebellar stimulation for
cerebral palsy spasticity, function, and
seizures. Archives of Medical Research.
2000;**31**(3):290-299

[140] Lin S et al. Superior cerebellar
peduncle deep brain stimulation for
cerebral palsy. Journal of Neurosurgery.
2024;**141**(5):1407-1417

[141] Harat M et al. Clinical evaluation
of deep cerebellar stimulation for
spasticity in patients with cerebral palsy.
Neurologia i Neurochirurgia Polska.
2009;**43**(1):36-44

[142] Lin S et al. High frequency deep
brain stimulation of superior cerebellar
peduncles in a patient with cerebral
palsy. Tremor and Other Hyperkinetic
Movements (New York, N.Y.).
2020;**10**:38

Chapter 3

Neurodevelopmental, Neurobehavioral, and Psychosocial Aspects of Cerebral Palsy

Ratnadeep Biswas

Abstract

Cerebral palsy (CP) is a group of permanent movement disorders caused by non-progressive disturbances in the developing brain. While motor impairments such as spasticity and dyskinesia are hallmark features, CP also encompasses the significant neurodevelopmental and neurobehavioral challenges. Cognitive deficits, ranging from mild intellectual disabilities to specific impairments in memory, attention, and executive functioning, are common and often exacerbated by comorbidities such as epilepsy or sensory impairments. Language and communication difficulties, including dysarthria and expressive-receptive language disorders, further hinder academic and social integration. Learning disabilities, compounded by motor and cognitive limitations, necessitate individualized educational plans and assistive technologies to support academic success. Behavioral comorbidities, such as attention-deficit/hyperactivity disorder (ADHD) and autism spectrum disorder (ASD), are prevalent in CP, complicating social interactions and academic progress. Management strategies include behavioral therapies such as applied behavior analysis and, when necessary, pharmacological interventions such as stimulant medications. Neurobehavioral assessments in CP are challenging due to motor and sensory impairments, requiring adapted tools and multidisciplinary collaboration for accurate evaluation. Psychosocial and emotional well-being is significantly impacted, with individuals often experiencing frustration, low self-esteem, and social isolation. Families also face emotional, financial, and social burdens, necessitating family-centered care approaches, including respite care, parent training programs, and support groups.

Keywords: cerebral palsy, neurodevelopmental disorders, cognition disorders, language disorders, learning disabilities, individualized education program, neuropsychological tests, quality of life

1. Introduction

Cerebral palsy (CP) is a heterogeneous group of permanent movement disorders that manifest in early childhood, stemming from non-progressive disturbances in the developing fetal or infant brain. These disturbances can occur prenatally, perinatally, or postnatally and are often associated with a wide range of etiologies, including pre-natal infections, birth complications, neonatal stroke, and genetic factors [1]. While CP is primarily defined by its motor impairments—such as spasticity, dyskinesia, or ataxia—it is increasingly recognized as a condition with multifaceted neurodevelop-mental and neurobehavioral implications [2]. These implications extend far beyond motor dysfunction, significantly influencing cognitive, linguistic, and learning abilities, as well as emotional and social functioning.

The neurodevelopmental and neurobehavioral challenges associated with CP are profound and pervasive. Cognitive deficits, which range from mild intellectual disabilities to specific impairments in executive functioning, memory, and attention, are common and can profoundly affect a child's ability to learn and interact with their environment. Language and communication difficulties, often exacerbated by motor speech disorders such as dysarthria, further compound these challenges, creating barriers to academic achievement and social integration. Additionally, learning dis-abilities, which may involve difficulties with reading, writing, and mathematics, are frequently observed in children with CP, necessitating tailored educational interven-tions and support systems [2].

Behavioral comorbidities, such as attention-deficit/hyperactivity disorder (ADHD) and autism spectrum disorder (ASD), are also prevalent in individuals with CP. These conditions not only exacerbate existing cognitive and social challenges but also introduce new layers of complexity to the management and care of affected individuals [3]. For instance, ADHD, characterized by inattention, hyperactivity, and impulsivity, can hinder academic progress and social interactions, while ASD, with its core deficits in social communication and repetitive behaviors, can further isolate children with CP from their peers. Understanding and addressing these behavioral comorbidities is critical for developing effective, holistic intervention strategies.

Conducting neurobehavioral assessments in individuals with CP presents unique challenges. Traditional assessment tools, which often rely on fine motor skills, verbal responses, or sustained attention, may not be suitable for children with significant motor or sensory impairments [4]. This can lead to underestimation of cognitive abilities and misdiagnosis of behavioral conditions. As a result, there is a pressing need for adapted and tailored evaluation tools that account for the physical and sen-sory limitations of individuals with CP. Collaborative, multidisciplinary approaches involving psychologists, speech therapists, occupational therapists, and educators are essential to ensure accurate and comprehensive assessments.

Beyond the individual, CP has far-reaching implications for the psychosocial and emotional well-being of both patients and their families. Children and adolescents with CP often face social isolation, low self-esteem, and emotional distress due to their physical and cognitive limitations [5]. These challenges can persist into adult-hood, affecting independence, employment, and quality of life. Families of children with CP also experience significant emotional, financial, and social burdens. Parents may grapple with stress, anxiety, and depression, while siblings may feel neglected or overwhelmed by the demands of caregiving [6]. Addressing these psychosocial challenges requires a family-centered care approach that prioritizes the needs and well-being of both the individual with CP and their support network.

This chapter aims to provide a comprehensive exploration of the neurodevelop-mental and neurobehavioral aspects of cerebral palsy. It will delve into the cogni-tive, language, and learning deficits commonly associated with CP, examining how cerebral injury impacts these domains and the resulting challenges in academic and social settings.

By integrating current research and clinical insights, this chapter seeks to provide a holistic understanding of the neurobehavioral challenges in cerebral palsy and to offer practical, evidence-based approaches to their management. Through this exploration, we aim to improve outcomes and enhance the quality of life for individuals with CP and their families, fostering resilience, independence, and inclusion in all aspects of life.

2. Cognitive deficits in cerebral palsy

2.1 Impact of cerebral injury on cognition

The specific location and extent of the brain injury are critical determinants of the cognitive outcomes in individuals with CP. For instance, injuries to the prefrontal cortex may impair executive functioning, while damage to the temporal or parietal lobes can affect language processing and spatial reasoning [7]. These cognitive deficits are not uniform; they vary widely depending on the nature and severity of the brain injury, leading to a spectrum of cognitive profiles in individuals with CP [8].

Cognitive deficits in CP can range from mild to severe and often encompass difficulties in attention, memory, executive functioning, and problem-solving skills [9].

Attention deficits, for example, may manifest as an inability to sustain focus on tasks or heightened distractibility, which can significantly impact learning and academic performance [10].

Memory impairments, particularly in working memory, can hinder the ability to retain and manipulate information, further complicating educational and daily living tasks [11].

Executive functioning deficits, which include challenges with planning, organization, and cognitive flexibility, are also common and can affect a child's ability to adapt to new situations or solve problems effectively [12].

Research has consistently shown that children with CP tend to exhibit lower IQ scores compared to their typically developing peers [13]. However, it is important to recognize that cognitive abilities in CP are highly variable. While some children may experience significant intellectual disabilities, others may have average or even above-average intelligence despite their motor impairments [14]. This variability underscores the complexity of CP as a condition and highlights the importance of avoiding generalizations about cognitive potential. For example, a child with severe spastic quadriplegia may have intact cognitive abilities, while a child with milder motor impairments may struggle with significant cognitive challenges.

The heterogeneity of cognitive profiles in CP is further influenced by the presence of comorbid conditions, such as epilepsy, sensory impairments, or behavioral disorders such as ADHD and ASD. These comorbidities can exacerbate cognitive difficulties, creating additional barriers to learning and social interaction [15]. For instance, children with CP and epilepsy may experience cognitive decline over time due to the cumulative effects of seizures on brain function [7]. Similarly, sensory impairments, such as hearing or vision loss, can limit access to environmental stimuli, further hindering cognitive development.

In conclusion, the impact of cerebral injury on cognition in individuals with CP is profound and multifaceted. The location and extent of the brain injury play a crucial role in determining cognitive outcomes, which can range from mild deficits to significant intellectual disabilities. However, the heterogeneity of cognitive profiles in CP underscores the need for individualized assessment and intervention strategies. By leveraging early intervention, adaptive assessment tools, and multidisciplinary approaches, it is possible to support the cognitive development of children with CP and help them reach their full potential [16].

2.2 Language and communication challenges

Language and communication difficulties are prevalent among individuals with CP, especially those with more pronounced motor impairments. These challenges often stem from a combination of the primary brain injury and the secondary effects of motor and sensory limitations [17, 18]. For instance, dysarthria, a motor speech disorder commonly associated with CP, can significantly impair speech clarity, making verbal communication laborious and sometimes unintelligible. This disorder arises from weakened or uncoordinated muscles involved in speech production, further complicating the ability to express oneself effectively [19].

Beyond motor speech disorders, children with CP frequently encounter broader language-related issues, including delays or disorders in both expressive and receptive language skills. Expressive language deficits may manifest as difficulties in forming sentences, using appropriate vocabulary, or conveying thoughts coherently, while receptive language challenges can hinder the understanding of spoken or written language [20]. These impairments not only affect academic performance but also impede social interactions, potentially leading to feelings of isolation or frustration. The cumulative impact on a child's quality of life underscores the importance of timely and targeted interventions.

Speech and language therapy plays a pivotal role in mitigating these challenges. By addressing these communication barriers proactively, caregivers and professionals can foster greater independence and improve the long-term prospects for individuals with CP [19].

2.3 Learning deficits and academic challenges

Learning challenges in children with CP are often complex and interconnected, stemming from a combination of cognitive, language, and motor impairments [21]. These difficulties can manifest in various academic domains, including reading, writing, and mathematics. For example, fine motor impairments may hinder handwriting, while cognitive or language delays can affect comprehension, problem-solving, and the ability to follow complex instructions [22]. Such barriers frequently result in academic underachievement, necessitating targeted interventions to help children reach their full potential.

To address these challenges, individualized education plans (IEPs) are widely utilized to tailor educational strategies to the specific needs of children with CP [23]. IEPs are designed to accommodate a child's unique strengths and weaknesses, incorporating modifications such as extended time for tests, simplified assignments, and the integration of assistive technologies like speech-to-text software or adaptive keyboards [24]. These tools not only facilitate learning but also empower children to participate more actively in classroom activities, fostering a sense of inclusion and confidence.

By addressing learning deficits through personalized and multidisciplinary approaches, children with CP can achieve meaningful academic progress and build a foundation for lifelong learning.

3. Behavioral characteristics and comorbidities

Behavioral challenges are a significant concern for individuals with CP, with ADHD and ASD being among the most frequently observed comorbidities [25]. These conditions can compound the existing physical and cognitive challenges associated with CP, necessitating tailored interventions to address their unique impact.

3.1 ADHD in cerebral palsy

Children with CP are at a heightened risk of developing ADHD, with prevalence rates estimated to be between 15% and as high as 40%, significantly higher than in the general population [3, 26]. ADHD in CP is typically characterized by symptoms of inattention, hyperactivity, and impulsivity, which can further complicate academic performance and social interactions. For instance, inattention may hinder a child's ability to focus during classroom activities, while hyperactivity and impulsivity can disrupt peer relationships and group tasks. These behavioral challenges often overlap with the motor and cognitive impairments of CP, creating a multifaceted barrier to learning and development. Early diagnosis and intervention, including behavioral therapy and, in some cases, medication, are essential for managing ADHD symptoms and improving functional outcomes [15, 27].

3.2 Autism spectrum disorder in cerebral palsy

Autism spectrum disorder is another common comorbidity in children with CP, with prevalence rates ranging from 6 to 8%, with odds roughly five times greater than those without CP [3, 28]. The co-occurrence of CP and ASD presents unique challenges, as the social communication deficits characteristics of ASD are often exacerbated by the motor and language impairments associated with CP. For example, a child with both conditions may struggle to use gestures or facial expressions to communicate, further isolating them from social interactions. Additionally, sensory processing issues, common in ASD, can be intensified by the physical limitations of CP, leading to heightened frustration or anxiety. Early identification of ASD in children with CP is critical, as it allows for the implementation of targeted interventions, such as social skills training and sensory integration therapy, to address these overlapping challenges [28].

3.3 Management strategies for behavioral challenges

Effectively addressing behavioral challenges in children with CP requires a multifaceted approach that combines therapeutic, educational, and, when necessary, pharmacological interventions. Given the high prevalence of these comorbidities, tailored strategies are essential to improve behavioral outcomes and enhance quality of life.

3.3.1 Behavioral therapy

Behavioral therapy is a cornerstone of managing behavioral challenges in children with CP, particularly for those with ADHD or ASD [29]. Applied behavior analysis (ABA) is one of the most widely used and evidence-based approaches. ABA focuses on teaching new skills, reducing problematic behaviors, and improving social interactions through structured, goal-oriented interventions [30, 31]. For example, ABA can help children with CP and ASD develop communication skills or reduce repetitive behaviors, while also addressing impulsivity and inattention in those with ADHD [32].

Parent training programs are another critical component of behavioral therapy. These programs equip parents with the tools and strategies needed to reinforce positive behaviors and manage challenging ones at home. By fostering consistency between therapy sessions and daily life, parent training enhances the effectiveness of behavioral interventions and supports long-term progress [32, 33].

3.3.2 Pharmacological interventions

In cases where behavioral therapy alone is insufficient, pharmacological interventions may be considered, particularly for children with CP and ADHD. Stimulant medications, such as methylphenidate, have been shown to effectively reduce symptoms of inattention, hyperactivity, and impulsivity in this population [34]. These medications can help children focus better in school, improve their ability to follow instructions, and enhance their overall functioning.

However, the use of stimulant medications requires careful monitoring due to potential side effects, such as decreased appetite, sleep disturbances, or increased anxiety. Healthcare providers must weigh the benefits and risks on an individual basis, ensuring that medication is part of a comprehensive treatment plan that includes behavioral and educational supports [35].

4. Neurobehavioral assessments in cerebral palsy

Assessing neurobehavioral functioning in individuals with CP is a complex process that requires careful consideration of the unique challenges posed by motor and sensory impairments. Traditional assessment tools often fall short in accurately capturing the cognitive, language, and behavioral abilities of children with CP, necessitating the use of adapted and multidisciplinary approaches.

4.1 Challenges in assessment

Conducting neurobehavioral assessments in children with CP is inherently difficult due to the interplay of motor, sensory, and communication impairments. Many standardized assessment tools rely on fine motor skills, verbal responses, or the ability to remain seated for prolonged periods—tasks that can be particularly challenging for children with CP. For instance, a child with severe spasticity may struggle to manipulate objects or point to answers, while a child with dysarthria may have difficulty providing verbal responses. These limitations can lead to an underestimation of cognitive abilities and result in inaccurate diagnoses or misclassification of developmental delays [4, 36].

4.2 Tailored evaluation tools

To overcome these challenges, researchers and clinicians have developed and adapted assessment tools specifically designed for children with CP. Instruments such as the Bayley Scales of Infant and Toddler Development (Bayley-III) and the Mullen Scales of Early Learning are widely used to evaluate developmental milestones in young children with CP [37, 38]. These tools have been modified to account for motor and sensory limitations, enabling a more accurate assessment of cognitive and language abilities. For example, alternative response methods, such as eye gaze or switch-activated devices, can be incorporated to accommodate children with severe physical impairments [39].

In addition to standardized assessments, qualitative measures play a crucial role in understanding a child's functioning in real-world contexts. Parent and teacher reports provide valuable insights into how the child performs in everyday settings, offering a more holistic view of their strengths and challenges. These reports can complement formal assessments by highlighting areas of need that may not be evident in a clinical setting [40, 41].

4.3 Collaborative assessment approaches

A comprehensive understanding of a child's neurobehavioral profile often requires input from a multidisciplinary team, including psychologists, speech therapists, occupational therapists, and educators. Collaborative assessments ensure that all aspects of the child's development are considered, from cognitive and language skills to social and emotional functioning. This team-based approach not only improves the accuracy of the assessment but also helps in developing individualized intervention plans that address the child's specific needs [42].

5. Psychosocial and emotional well-being

The psychosocial and emotional well-being of individuals with CP is profoundly influenced by the neurodevelopmental and neurobehavioral challenges associated with the condition. These challenges can affect not only the individuals themselves but also their families, creating a ripple effect that necessitates comprehensive support systems and interventions [43].

5.1 Impact on patients

Children with CP often face significant emotional and psychosocial challenges due to their physical and cognitive limitations. Feelings of frustration, low self-esteem, and social isolation are common, particularly when communication or mobility barriers hinder their ability to participate in social activities or achieve age-appropriate milestones [44]. The presence of comorbid conditions, such as ADHD or ASD, can further compound these difficulties, leading to heightened emotional distress and behavioral challenges.

As individuals with CP transition into adolescence and adulthood, they may encounter additional psychosocial hurdles. These can include difficulties in securing employment, establishing independent living arrangements, and navigating social relationships. The transition to adulthood is often particularly challenging, as support systems that were available during childhood may no longer be accessible. Mental health support, including counseling and psychotherapy, plays a critical role in addressing these challenges, helping individuals build resilience and improve their emotional well-being [45].

5.2 Impact on families

The emotional, financial, and social burdens of caring for a child with CP can significantly impact families. Parents often experience high levels of stress, anxiety, and depression, particularly when they face challenges in accessing appropriate services or balancing caregiving responsibilities with other life demands [46]. Siblings of children with CP may also be affected, as they may feel neglected or overwhelmed by the additional attention and resources directed toward their sibling with a disability. These dynamics can strain family relationships and disrupt the overall family equilibrium [47].

5.3 Family-centered care and support strategies

Family-centered care is a cornerstone of effective CP management, emphasizing the importance of involving families in decision-making processes and providing holistic support. This approach recognizes that the well-being of the child with CP is closely tied to the well-being of their family. Collaborative care models, which involve healthcare providers, educators, and families working together, have been shown to improve outcomes for the child while also enhancing the emotional and social health of the entire family.

Support strategies for families may include access to respite care, which offers temporary relief for caregivers, allowing them to recharge and attend to their own needs. Parent training programs, such as the Stepping Stones Triple P (Positive Parenting Program), equip parents with practical strategies for managing their child's behavior and fostering positive family interactions [48]. Additionally, support groups—both in-person and online—provide families with a sense of community, enabling them to share experiences, resources, and coping strategies [49, 50].

6. Conclusions

Cerebral palsy is a complex condition that encompasses a wide range of neurodevelopmental and neurobehavioral challenges. Cognitive, language, and learning deficits are common in individuals with CP and can significantly impact academic achievement and social interaction. Behavioral challenges, such as ADHD and autism, are also prevalent and require tailored management strategies, including behavioral therapy and pharmacological interventions.

Conducting neurobehavioral assessments in individuals with CP can be challenging due to motor and sensory impairments, highlighting the need for tailored evaluation tools. The psychosocial and emotional well-being of both patients and families is a critical consideration, and family-centered care approaches are essential for providing comprehensive support.

This chapter has provided a comprehensive overview of the neurobehavioral challenges in cerebral palsy and evidence-based approaches to their management. By addressing these challenges through individualized assessment, intervention, and support, we can improve outcomes and enhance the quality of life for individuals with CP and their families.

Acknowledgements

I thank the readers for their time and sincerely hope that this chapter offers meaningful insights into the diverse neurodevelopmental and neurobehavioral dimensions of cerebral palsy.

Conflict of interest

The author declares no conflicts of interest.

Appendixes and nomenclature

CP	cerebral palsy
ADHD	attention-deficit/hyperactivity disorder
ASD	autism spectrum disorder
IEPs	individualized education plans
ABA	applied behavior analysis

Author details

Ratnadeep Biswas
All India Institute of Medical Sciences, Patna, India

*Address all correspondence to: ratnadeepbis2404@gmail.com

IntechOpen

References

[1] Hallman-Cooper JL, Rocha CF. Cerebral Palsy. StatPearls, Treasure Island (FL): StatPearls Publishing; 2025

[2] Patel DR, Neelakantan M, Pandher K, Merrick J. Cerebral palsy in children: A clinical overview. Translational Pediatrics. 2020;**9**:S125-S135. DOI: 10.21037/tp.2020.01.01

[3] Chen Q, Chen M, Bao W, Strathearn L, Zang X, Meng L, et al. Association of cerebral palsy with autism spectrum disorder and attention-deficit/hyperactivity disorder in children: A large-scale nationwide population-based study. BMJ Paediatrics Open. 2024;**8**:e002343. DOI: 10.1136/bmjpo-2023-002343

[4] Javvaji CK, Vagha JD, Meshram RJ, Taksande A. Assessment scales in cerebral palsy: A comprehensive review of tools and applications. Cureus. n.d.;**15**:e47939. DOI: 10.7759/cureus.47939

[5] Cheshire A, Barlow JH, Powell LA. The psychosocial well-being of parents of children with cerebral palsy: A comparison study. Disability and Rehabilitation. 2010;**32**:1673-1677. DOI: 10.3109/09638281003649920

[6] Vadivelan K, Sekar P, Sruthi SS, Gopichandran V. Burden of caregivers of children with cerebral palsy: An intersectional analysis of gender, poverty, stigma, and public policy. BMC Public Health. 2020;**20**:645. DOI: 10.1186/s12889-020-08808-0

[7] Bottcher L. Children with spastic cerebral palsy, their cognitive functioning, and social participation: A review. Child Neuropsychology. 2010;**16**:209-228. DOI: 10.1080/09297040903559630

[8] Anderson V, Spencer-Smith M, Wood A. Do children really recover better? Neurobehavioural plasticity after early brain insult. Brain. 2011;**134**:2197-2221. DOI: 10.1093/brain/awr103

[9] Stadskleiv K, Jahnsen R, Andersen GL, Von Tetzchner S. Neuropsychological profiles of children with cerebral palsy. Developmental Neurorehabilitation. 2018;**21**:108-120. DOI: 10.1080/17518423.2017.1282054

[10] Students Experiencing Inattention and Distractibility. Available from: https://www.apa.org/ed/schools/primer/inattention [Accessed: January 31, 2025]

[11] Cowan N. Working memory underpins cognitive development, learning, and education. Educational Psychology Review. 2014;**26**:197-223. DOI: 10.1007/s10648-013-9246-y

[12] Jacobson LA, Williford AP, Pianta RC. The role of executive function in children's competent adjustment to middle school. Child Neuropsychology: A Journal on Normal and Abnormal Development in Childhood and Adolescence. 2011;**17**:255-280. DOI: 10.1080/09297049.2010.535654

[13] Yin Foo R, Guppy M, Johnston LM. Intelligence assessments for children with cerebral palsy: A systematic review. Developmental Medicine and Child Neurology. 2013;**55**:911-918. DOI: 10.1111/dmcn.12157

[14] Sigurdardottir S, Eiriksdottir A, Gunnarsdottir E, Meintema M, Arnadottir U, Vik T. Cognitive profile in young Icelandic children with cerebral palsy. Developmental Medicine and Child Neurology. 2008;**50**:357-362. DOI: 10.1111/j.1469-8749.2008.02046.x

[15] Craig F, Savino R, Trabacca A. A systematic review of comorbidity between cerebral palsy, autism spectrum disorders and attention deficit hyperactivity disorder. European Journal of Paediatric Neurology. 2019;**23**:31-42. DOI: 10.1016/j.ejpn.2018.10.005

[16] Damiano DL, Longo E. Early intervention evidence for infants with or at risk for cerebral palsy: An overview of systematic reviews. Developmental Medicine and Child Neurology. 2021;**63**:771-784. DOI: 10.1111/dmcn.14855

[17] Mineo BA. Communication in Children and Youth with Cerebral Palsy. In: Miller F, Bachrach S, Lennon N, O'Neil ME, editors. Cerebral Palsy. Cham: Springer International Publishing; 2020. pp. 2883-2902. DOI: 10.1007/978-3-319-74558-9_177

[18] Fluss J, Lidzba K. Cognitive and academic profiles in children with cerebral palsy: A narrative review. Annals of Physical and Rehabilitation Medicine. 2020;**63**:447-456. DOI: 10.1016/j.rehab.2020.01.005

[19] Pennington L, Goldbart J, Marshall J. Speech and language therapy to improve the communication skills of children with cerebral palsy. Cochrane Database of Systematic Reviews. 2004;**2004**:CD003466. DOI: 10.1002/14651858.CD003466.pub2

[20] Hustad KC, Gorton K, Lee J. Classification of speech and language profiles in 4-year-old children with cerebral palsy: A prospective preliminary study. Journal of Speech, Language, and Hearing Research. 2010;**53**:1496-1513. DOI: 10.1044/1092-4388(2010/09-0176)

[21] Morgan P, McGinley JL. Cerebral palsy. In: Day BL, Lord SR, editors. Handbook of Clinical Neurology. Vol. 159. Elsevier; 2018. pp. 323-336. DOI: 10.1016/B978-0-444-63916-5.00020-3

[22] Fauconnier J, Dickinson HO, Beckung E, Marcelli M, McManus V, Michelsen SI, et al. Participation in life situations of 8-12 year old children with cerebral palsy: Cross sectional European study. BMJ. 2009;**338**:b1458. DOI: 10.1136/bmj.b1458

[23] Samiuddin Z, Naser Z. Effectiveness of IEPs (Individual Education Plans) for Children with Diverse Learning Needs and Abilities (an Exploratory Study). Islamabad, Pakistan: Virtual University; 2022. DOI: 10.13140/RG.2.2.11797.50402

[24] Rosenbaum P, Paneth N, Leviton A, Goldstein M, Bax M, Damiano D, et al. A report: The definition and classification of cerebral palsy April 2006. Developmental Medicine and Child Neurology. Supplement. 2007;**109**:8-14

[25] van Steensel FJA, Bögels SM, de Bruin EI. Psychiatric comorbidity in children with autism spectrum disorders: A comparison with children with ADHD. Journal of Child and Family Studies. 2013;**22**:368-376. DOI: 10.1007/s10826-012-9587-z

[26] Shank LK, Kaufman J, Leffard S, Warschausky S. Inspection time and ADHD symptoms in children with cerebral palsy. Rehabilitation Psychology. 2010;**55**:188-193. DOI: 10.1037/a0019601

[27] Lidzba K, Granström S, Lindenau J, Mautner V. The adverse influence of attention-deficit disorder with or without hyperactivity on cognition in neurofibromatosis type 1. Developmental Medicine and Child Neurology. 2012;**54**:892-897. DOI: 10.1111/j.1469-8749.2012.04377.x

[28] Casseus M, Shoval HA, Erasmus AJ, Cheng J. Clinical and functional

characteristics of co-occurring cerebral palsy and autism spectrum disorder among children and young adults. Research in Autism Spectrum Disorder. 2024;**118**:102490. DOI: 10.1016/j.rasd.2024.102490

[29] Behavioral Management Therapy for Autism | NICHD - Eunice Kennedy Shriver National Institute of Child Health and Human Development n.d. Available from:https://www.nichd.nih.gov/health/topics/autism/conditioninfo/treatments/behavioral-management [Accessed: January 31, 2025]

[30] Slocum TA, Detrich R, Wilczynski SM, Spencer TD, Lewis T, Wolfe K. The evidence-based practice of applied behavior analysis. Behavior Analyst. 2014;**37**:41-56. DOI: 10.1007/s40614-014-0005-2

[31] Du G, Guo Y, Xu W. The effectiveness of applied behavior analysis program training on enhancing autistic children's emotional-social skills. BMC Psychology. 2024;**12**:568. DOI: 10.1186/s40359-024-02045-5

[32] Silberg T, Kapil N, Caven I, Levac D, Fehlings D. Cognitive behavioral therapies for individuals with cerebral palsy: A scoping review. Developmental Medicine and Child Neurology. 2023;**65**:1012-1028. DOI: 10.1111/dmcn.15507

[33] Reichow B, Barton EE, Boyd BA, Hume K. Early intensive behavioral intervention (EIBI) for young children with autism spectrum disorders (ASD). Cochrane Database of Systematic Reviews. 2012;**2018**(5):1-52, CD009260. DOI: 10.1002/14651858.CD009260.pub2

[34] Sibley MH, Bruton AM, Zhao X, Johnstone JM, Mitchell J, Hatsu I, et al. Non-pharmacological interventions for attention-deficit hyperactivity disorder in children and adolescents. The Lancet Child & Adolescent Health. 2023;**7**:415-428. DOI: 10.1016/S2352-4642(22)00381-9

[35] Shrestha M, Lautenschleger J, Soares N. Non-pharmacologic management of attention-deficit/hyperactivity disorder in children and adolescents: A review. Translational Pediatrics. 2020;**9**:S114-S124. DOI: 10.21037/tp.2019.10.01

[36] Twum F, Hayford JK. Motor development in cerebral palsy and its relationship to intellectual development: A review article. European Journal of Medical and Health Sciences. 2024;**6**:8-15. DOI: 10.24018/ejmed.2024.6.5.2161

[37] Balasundaram P, Avulakunta ID. Bayley Scales of Infant and Toddler Development. StatPearls, Treasure Island (FL): StatPearls Publishing; 2025

[38] Burns TG, King TZ, Spencer KS. Mullen scales of early learning: The utility in assessing children diagnosed with autism spectrum disorders, cerebral palsy, and epilepsy. Applied Neuropsychology: Child. 2013;**2**:33-42. DOI: 10.1080/21622965.2012.682852

[39] Pa O, Johnston C, VLJ K, RPV F, WB C. Assessment of child development by the Bayley III scale: A systematic review. Clinical Case Reports are fully Open Access. 2022;**5**. DOI: 10.46527/2582-5038.205

[40] Cerebral Palsy General Assessment. Physiopedia n.d. Available from: https://www.physio-pedia.com/Cerebral_Palsy_General_Assessment [Accessed: January 31, 2025]

[41] Kumar S. Impact of Assessment on childhood education theories and practice. In: Badea M, Suditu M, editors. The Advances in Early Childhood and K-12 Education. Educ: IGI Global;

2024. pp. 84-101. DOI: 10.4018/979-8-
3693-0956-8.ch004

[42] Ogundele MO. A multidisciplinary
approach to the assessment and
management of pre-school age Neurodevelopmental disorders: A local
experience. Clinical Journal of Nursing
Care and Practice. 2017;**1**:001-012.
DOI: 10.29328/journal.cjncp.1001001

[43] Williams C, Wood RL, Alderman N,
Worthington A. The psychosocial impact
of neurobehavioral disability. Frontiers
in Neurology. 2020;**11**:119. DOI: 10.3389/
fneur.2020.00119

[44] Brossard-Racine M, Hall N,
Majnemer A, Shevell MI, Law M, Poulin C,
et al. Behavioural problems in school
age children with cerebral palsy. The
European Journal of Paediatric Neurology
is the Official Journal of the European
Paediatric Neurology Society. 2012;**16**:35-
41. DOI: 10.1016/j.ejpn.2011.10.001

[45] Young N, McCormick A, Mills W,
Barden W, Boydell K, Law M, et al. The
transition study: A look at youth and
adults with cerebral palsy, spina bifida
and acquired brain injury. Physical &
Occupational Therapy in Pediatrics.
2006;**26**:25-45

[46] Raina P, O'Donnell M, Rosenbaum P,
Brehaut J, Walter SD, Russell D, et al. The
health and well-being of caregivers of
children with cerebral palsy. Pediatrics.
2005;**115**:e626-e636. DOI: 10.1542/
peds.2004-1689

[47] Dias BLS, de Rodrigues MCC,
Duarte JLMB. Quality of life of
families and siblings of children with
cerebral palsy treated at a reference
neurorehabilitation center in Brazil.
Jornal de Pediatria. 2024;**100**:519-526.
DOI: 10.1016/j.jped.2024.03.010

[48] Whittingham K, Wee D,
Sanders MR, Boyd R. Predictors of

psychological adjustment, experienced
parenting burden and chronic sorrow
symptoms in parents of children with
cerebral palsy. Child: Care, Health
and Development. 2013;**39**:366-373.
DOI: 10.1111/j.1365-2214.2012.01396.x

[49] Cerebral Palsy Support Groups
and Organizations. Cereb Palsy Guid.
n.d. Available from: https://www.
cerebralpalsyguidance.com/cerebral-
palsy/support-groups/ [Accessed:
January 31, 2025]

[50] Chakraborti M, Gitimoghaddam M,
McKellin WH, Miller AR, Collet J-P.
Understanding the implications of peer
support for families of children with
neurodevelopmental and intellectual
disabilities: A scoping review. Frontiers
in Public Health. 2021;**9**:719640.
DOI: 10.3389/fpubh.2021.719640

Chapter 4

Influence of Robotic Interventions on Gait Improvement in Children with Cerebral Palsy

Lihua Jin, Caixia Zhao, Binjing Dou, Juchuan Dong and Ping He

Abstract

For individuals with cerebral palsy (CP), walking ability is of critical importance, as highlighted by the focus on gross motor function within their primary outcome measure, the Gross Motor Function Classification System (GMFCS). This focus underscores the intricate connection between walking ability and participation, activity, and physical function. Despite extensive and prolonged therapeutic interventions, rehabilitation efforts often fail to produce significant improvements in walking ability for individuals with CP. Recently, robotic-assisted gait training (RAGT) has emerged as a promising therapeutic modality for enhancing walking capabilities in this population. RAGT offers the potential for personalized interventions by adjusting parameters such as assistance level, resistance, and body weight support to cater to the specific needs of individuals with CP. Nevertheless, the evidence supporting the efficacy of RAGT remains limited. This chapter comprehensively reviews the challenges associated with walking in individuals with CP, explores the potential benefits and various forms of RAGT, and discusses future research directions.

Keywords: cerebral palsy, robotic-assisted gait training, physical therapy, neurorehabilitation, motorskills

1. Introduction

Cerebral palsy (CP), caused by brain damage prenatally, perinatally, or postnatally, is the most common cause of childhood movement and posture-related disability. Motor impairments manifest in approximately 80% of children with CP, resulting in secondary complications such as hip pain, dislocation, balance issues, hand dysfunction, and equinus deformity [1]. The brain damage associated with CP can result in positive symptoms, including muscle spasms and hypertonia, and/or negative symptoms, such as muscle weakness, loss of motor control, muscle wasting, and impaired balance reactions. The predominant motor disorders associated with CP include spasticity and abnormalities in muscle tone, which are commonly associated with challenges in coordination, strength, and selective motor control. These conditions can result in spasticity-induced deformities of the bones and joints, as well as pain and functional impairment [2]. Muscle injuries arising from spasms, weakness, abnormal tone, or pain can further diminish joint range of motion and selective motor control. Consequently, difficulties regulating the flexion angles of the lower limb joints, specifically the hip, knee, and ankle, impede the ambulatory capabilities of affected children, thereby impacting on daily activities. Gait abnormalities, including crouch gait, toe walking, and scissoring, are frequently observed in children with CP and are often linked to diminished participation in daily activities and social interactions, underscoring the importance of maintaining and enhancing walking ability through-out all stages of CP management.

Abnormal gait associated with CP can present in various forms, which are pre-dominantly categorized as pathological gait patterns. For example, individuals with spastic CP display a reduction in the muscle volume of the gastrocnemius and tibialis anterior, accompanied by an increased echo intensity, indicative of abnormal ankle gait characteristics [3]. Patients with CP also exhibit a reduced number of muscle synergies during gait, indicating the adoption of a simplified control strategy during ambula-tion, potentially linked to diminished neuromuscular control complexity. Among younger patients with CP, the most prevalent gait abnormality is true equinus gait [4]. At this developmental stage, the patient's body weight is relatively low, and the muscle strength of the hip and knee joints remains robust; however, plantar flexion is caused by the shortening of the gastrocnemius muscle group. This abnormal gait is character-ized by forefoot contact during the stance phase, with normal flexion and extension of the hip and knee joints. As patients with CP age, their body weight increases, concurrent with the shortening or weakening of the proximal muscles. This results in significant flexion of the hip and knee joints during the single-stance phase, resulting in a gait pattern that resembles a jump. As this proximal muscle weakness progresses, supporting the body weight becomes increasingly complicated, resulting in a more pronounced flexion of the hip and knee joints, leading to the development of a distinct equinus gait. Eventually, when patients with CP experience dorsiflexion of the foot and ankle, along with severe flexion of the hip and knee joints, the gait transitions into a crouch gait. Crouch gait, the ultimate developmental stage of gait dysfunction in these patients, is also the prevalent gait abnormality observed in children with CP [5]. These disparate gait patterns all develop as compensatory mechanisms for insufficient muscle strength to support body weight. However, all are unsustainable and tend to deteriorate as the patient grows and gains weight, ultimately resulting in a loss of motor function. Consequently, it is imperative to devise strategies aimed at maintaining long-term gait function to enhance the rehabilitation outcomes of patients with CP.

In this chapter, we discuss the use of robotic-assisted gait training (RAGT) as the potential intervention in the improvement of locomotor function in patients with CP.

2. Gait enhancement strategies in children with CP

Due to the heterogeneous nature of CP, patients with CP exhibit a diverse array of associated challenges and motor impairments that necessitate evaluation and intervention by a multidisciplinary team of specialists. Enhancing gait is a critical therapeutic objective in CP management; however, conventional gait rehabilitation methods are often unsustainable for patients. While early initiation of rehabilita-tion, particularly through a combination of physical and occupational therapy, may enhance outcomes [6], conventional rehabilitation approaches have demonstrated limited efficacy in the treatment of CP. This limitation is especially pertinent given that rehabilitation largely depends on the brain's neuroplasticity, which tends to be less responsive to interventions in adult individuals with CP [7]. Notably, adults with CP may derive cardiovascular benefits from physical therapy interventions, such as aerobic exercise and resistance training; however, significant improvements in walking ability are unlikely to be achieved [8]. Other potential strategies include surgical interventions, whose effects are often transient, losing efficacy as children grow and develop, and manual assistance, which is limited by its demanding, intensive, and continuous nature. Robotic technology is an innovative rehabilitation approach that employs computer-controlled systems to facilitate motor learning and cortical reorganization, thereby enhancing limb function.

3. An introduction to RAGT

Prior studies have shown that gait rehabilitation incorporating functional movements has greater efficacy than training employing nonfunctional movement patterns. RAGT offers precise and intensive task-specific training, while simultaneously collecting data from multiple sensors to accurately capture patient information, such as limb kinematics, kinetics, electromyography (EMG) pattern, electroencephalography (EEG) patterns, and energy expenditure, during practice. Thus, the implementation of robotic-assisted therapy has the potential to alleviate skilled therapists from the physical demands associated with direct hands-on therapy. Furthermore, RAGT offers repetitive, continuous, graded, and task-specific training aimed at improving gait function by establishing conditions conducive to motor learning principles, such as intensity, repetition, task specificity, and engagement. As such, this rehabilitation strategy facilitates neuroplastic changes and enhances non-locomotor recovery in children with CP experiencing movement disorders of a central origin.

Repetitive RAGT fosters functional network reorganization within the sensorimotor cortex and stimulates neuroplasticity [9] while enhancing functional connectivity between the frontal and parietal regions [10]. The mechanisms by which RAGT influences the brain are intricate, involving multiple neural pathways and cortical regions. Early initiation of RAGT following brain injury can markedly expedite the bilateral reorganization of motor-related brain areas [11]. Studies employing functional near-infrared spectroscopy (fNIRS) to monitor changes in the cerebral cortex during RAGT have revealed that prompt RAGT intervention can significantly enhance cortical activation associated with motor control; indeed, this activation extends beyond the motor areas to encompass various functional brain regions [12]. Furthermore, RAGT has the potential to modulate the overall efficiency of brain networks, facilitating the restoration of normal brain network organization, and thereby promoting functional recovery [13]. Together, these findings indicate that RAGT holds significant potential for improving motor function and quality of life among children with CP.

RAGT integrates exoskeleton technology with information control systems to aid in human movement through precise mechanical devices. This approach necessitates interdisciplinary expertise, encompassing biomechanics, robotics, information science, and artificial intelligence. Typically, these robotic systems are outfitted with sensors capable of performing real-time, high-precision assessments of patients' rehabilitation status, including metrics such as joint range of motion, force output, walking speed, and step length. Furthermore, these systems can autonomously adapt to each patient, based on individual data, thereby allowing the personalization of rehabilitation programs [14].

4. Forms of RAGT

Functionally, RAGT can be categorized into two primary types: traction-type and exoskeleton-type. The defining characteristic of traction-type RAGT is its ability to facilitate the training of the hip, knee, and ankle joints by directing movement of the patient's feet. The end-effector traction-type robot does not require alignment of its hardware system with the patient's joint structure, thereby enhancing its user-friendliness. Consequently, this type of rehabilitation robot is recognized for its high safety standards during training sessions. In contrast, exoskeleton-type RAGT is characterized by a more intricate structure with advanced functionalities and capabilities. Compared to traction-type robots, exoskeleton-type can interpret each patient's movement intentions, simulating and controlling multiple joints based on normal gait patterns, thereby offering personalized support. Consequently, exoskeleton-type RAGT is regarded as an emerging research direction and developmental trend within the rehabilitation domain.

RAGT integrates bilateral robotic orthoses, body weight support (BWS), and a treadmill. As a computerized system, it allows for the adjustment of BWS to ensure an upright posture and precise lower limb loading. The orthoses used in RAGT facilitate leg movements within the sagittal plane, following repeatable, pre-defined trajectories of the hip and knee joints. Simultaneously, footplates maintain passive ankle dorsiflexion, thereby assisting individuals with CP in performing ambulation. RAGT offers a controlled and safe therapeutic environment, enabling patients to participate in prolonged training sessions through numerous repetitions of steps while promoting repeatable, kinematically consistent symmetrical gait patterns [15].

5. Clinical utility of RAGT

The most commonly employed form of RAGT in clinical practice involves the use of tethered exoskeleton systems, which exert force through a rigid, articulated frame that facilitates the movement of the patient's legs across one or more planes *via* a body weight support system [16], such as the Lokomat (Hocoma AG, Volketswil, Switzerland) system. Nevertheless, current supporting evidence remains insufficient to demonstrate that these systems yield superior therapeutic outcomes in terms of gross motor function and walking ability compared with conventional physiotherapy [17]. The primary limitation of these systems includes their reliance on predetermined fixed trajectories or timings, which restricts the patient's active participation consequently diminishing muscle activity. Furthermore, when patients attempt to walk actively and resist the device, abnormal muscle activation patterns may develop [18]. In contrast, untethered exoskeletons, such as ReWalk (ReWalk Robotics Inc., Marlborough, MA, USA), Indego (Parker Hannifin Corp, Mayfield Heights, OH, USA), Hybrid Assistive Limb (HAL, Cyberdyne Inc., Tsukuba, Japan), and Ekso (Ekso Bionics, Richmond, CA, USA), are wearable systems comprising articulated suits that are self-powered and equipped with advanced control algorithms. These systems, which are used for gait assistance and rehabilitation, provide task-specific overground training to offer patients a more liberated and realistic walking experience.

6. Clinically available RAGT devices

Various RAGT devices offer stability and partial body weight support for pediatric patients engaged in overground walking training. By enabling the individualized control of each joint, these devices can operate in multiple modes, including position control, resistance, and zero-force control, thereby allowing movements to be tailored to each patient's current capabilities and enhancing the system's modularity [19], as exemplified by devices such as the CP Walker. The Innowalk Pro (IP) [20] is a standing apparatus designed to facilitate movement across different spatial dimensions. This device adjusts the child's range of motion, frequency, and functionality during use to optimize therapeutic outcomes [21]. The Walkbot-K system includes both adult and pediatric exoskeleton RAGT models, with the pediatric version specifically designed for children with CP. This device can automatically adjust leg length to fit the child, thereby promoting functional improvement, while providing real-time assessments of muscle tone, muscle strength, and gait [22]. The pediatric knee exoskeleton (P.REX) is the second prototype of a tethered knee exoskeleton; the P.REX comprises an untethered device capable of delivering consistent knee extension torque throughout various movement phases [23]. The Honda Walking Assist (HWA) device, a wearable exoskeleton robot developed by Honda R&D Co., Ltd., was designed to facilitate bilateral hip flexion and extension during ambulation. Notably, the HWA targets a single joint without constraining the degrees of freedom of other joints, thereby permitting a high degree of movement and enhancing motor learning efficacy. HWA has been shown to significantly reduce energy expenditure in healthy young adults and can improve hip kinematic symmetry and step length in individuals with hemiparesis. Considering that the majority of children with CP exhibit bilateral neurological involvement and complicated lower limb symptoms, the HWA holds potential to aid these children in acquiring symmetrical gait patterns by supporting bilateral hip movements [20].

7. Clinical evidence supporting the utility of RAGT

Numerous studies investigating RAGT in populations with CP have employed systems using tethered exoskeletons, reporting consequent enhancements in gait speed, endurance, and gross motor function [24]. However, meta-analytical evaluations have deemed these findings statistically insignificant. A recent systematic review has highlighted that the evidence supporting the efficacy of RAGT for children with gait disorders, particularly CP, remains weak and inconsistent, with RAGT not demonstrating superior outcomes compared to traditional physical therapy [25]. Additional research has shown that RAGT does not significantly enhance standing ability or gait function in patients with CP classified as levels III to IV on the Gross Motor Function Classification System (GMFCS) [26]. Additionally, when motor function levels were not taken into account, randomized controlled trials assessing gait training interventions in patients with CP indicated that RAGT did not demonstrate superiority over conventional physical therapy [27]. Furthermore, studies have indicated that the harness-provided weight support and treadmill belt movement may render RAGT training more demanding and intense than overground walking [28]. Finally, the observed improvements in gait function may not translate effectively to overground walking, as treadmill training lacks task specificity for real-world environments.

In addition to RAGT application as a standalone intervention, promising outcomes have been observed for the combination of RAGT with other therapeutic modalities. For example, the integration of RAGT with botulinum toxin A (BoNT-A) enhanced gross motor function measure scores in children with CP, although RAGT did not amplify the anti-spasticity effects of BoNT-A. Nevertheless, its adjunctive use resulted in significant improvements in motor skills and gait in this population [29]. The combination of RAGT with virtual reality (VR) has further been reported to increase patient engagement and enjoyment during training, thereby effectively enhancing gait in children with CP [30]. Furthermore, RAGT in conjunction with noninvasive brain stimulation (NIBS) has shown the potential to improve lower limb function in various neurological populations [31]. Specifically, the combination of RAGT with repetitive transcranial magnetic stimulation (rTMS) can modulate cortical motor inhibition, resulting in gait improvements [32]. Additionally, the use of RAGT along-side transcranial direct current stimulation (tDCS) enhances balance and functional performance in individuals with CP [33].

Despite some skepticism, the beneficial effects of RAGT on various bodily functions in patients with CP cannot be dismissed. These benefits include improvements in joint range of motion [34–36], muscle tone [35]. muscle strength [34], balance [26], and short-term and long-term gait parameters, particularly gait speed [37]. Additionally, enhancements in gross motor function [26], particularly in patients classified as GMFCS levels IV and V, gait kinematics [38, 39], reduced metabolic cost during walking [40], and improved motor performance and endurance [16] have been observed. RAGT facilitates task-oriented repetitive movements, muscle strengthening, and motor coordination, all of which positively influence energy efficiency, gait speed, and balance control [41]. Given that long-term motor functional impairments can result in psychological issues, such as anxiety and depression, which may further exacerbate physical motor function, the efficacy of interventions targeting mental health is critical in the rehabilitation process. RAGT has been shown to enhance psychological well-being in patients with neurological impairments and positively affect short-term depressive symptoms.

The variability in RAGT outcomes between disparate studies may be attributed to differences in parameter settings, as RAGT combined with virtual reality achieved enhanced efficacy at improving BWS when body weight was reduced by 30% [30]. Additionally, the efficacy of RAGT may be influenced by the training mode employed. For example, the motor and constraint-induced movement therapy (CIMT) modes were more effective at enhancing balance and gait [42]. The intensity and frequency of RAGT are critical determinants of rehabilitation outcomes, which may directly impact alterations in patients' motor function. Tailoring the intensity of RAGT based on the GMFCS level presents a promising intervention strategy, as higher-intensity training has shown more substantial effects in individuals classified at GMFCS levels II and III. However, prior studies on RAGT have employed diverse training protocols and implemented differing procedures, complicating the comparison of results across studies. This heterogeneity in training protocols may have contributed to the limited clinical evidence supporting RAGT. Nevertheless, compared to other robotic interventions, such as patient-guided suspension systems and end-effector devices, RAGT has been shown to offer comprehensive control over leg joint angles and torques, making it the preferred robotic solution for training patients with severe motor impairments due to brain injury [43].

8. Integration of RAGT with additional interventional modalities

Within conventional rehabilitation frameworks, RAGT is frequently integrated with traditional physical therapy techniques, such as joint and muscle relaxation exercises, to improve joint flexibility. These exercises may be administered either prior to or following RAGT to enhance the therapeutic outcomes of both physical therapy and RAGT. This combined approach has been shown to consistently increase lower limb muscle strength, mitigate muscle atrophy, and enhance muscle endurance in patients. Additionally, the concurrent use of RAGT with pharmacological interventions is prevalent in clinical settings, particularly as patients with CP often require ongoing oral medications, including antiepileptics and muscle relaxants. The administration of these medications during RAGT sessions can enhance safety and improve patient adherence to RAGT movement protocols, thereby augmenting the efficacy of the training. In addition to the interventions outlined in Section 7 that can be integrated with RAGT, the RAGT apparatus itself, when equipped with training modules, offers potential benefits for patients with central nervous system injuries. For example, beyond the conventional linear walking patterns associated with traditional RAGT, the incorporation of motion capture devices for multi-directional tracking—including left, right, and bilateral multi-stage trajectories—can accommodate patients at various stages of injury recovery [44]. Furthermore, the integration of RAGT with acupuncture therapy may offer promise, potentially assisting patients with abnormal gait and walking difficulties [45]. With advancements in Transcutaneous Spinal Cord Stimulation (tSCS) technology, its combined application with RAGT has demonstrated improvements in gait-related parameters for patients with CP, such as enhanced upright posture and reduced crouching [46]. Nevertheless, the empirical support for these adjunctive treatment methods remains limited. Electromyography (EMG), when integrated with RAGT, emerges as a promising auxiliary instrument for assessing the origins of abnormal postures during gait interventions and for informing clinical decisions on targeted combined approaches [47]. However, the technical complexity of EMG poses significant challenges to its widespread application in clinical settings. Consequently, further investigation is warranted to identify more feasible enhancements for RAGT modules and its combined approaches to improve therapeutic efficacy.

9. Accessibility of RAGT

In recent years, RAGT has been increasingly investigated for its application in pediatric rehabilitation within several advanced nations, yielding significant outcomes that affirm its technical feasibility, clinical efficacy, and potential for promising development. The global exchange of medical technology has facilitated opportunities for the introduction of RAGT equipment in developing countries. International medical aid initiatives and charitable organizations may contribute to this effort by donating or funding the acquisition of RAGT equipment for health-care facilities in these regions, thereby progressively improving local accessibility. Although certain developing countries have endeavored to independently design and adapt RAGT equipment, achieving therapeutic benefits for patients with cerebral palsy [48, 49], the high costs associated with RAGT equipment and its maintenance, coupled with the operational complexity and requirement for specialized personnel, constrain its widespread adoption in grassroots hospitals and less developed regions [50]. Furthermore, the unequal distribution of treatment resources, particularly for rehabilitation technologies such as RAGT that necessitate substantial financial and technical investment, exacerbates existing regional disparities [51]. One approach to mitigating this disparity involves developing specialized expertise to serve regional populations using shared resources.

10. Conclusion

In summary, although significant strides have been made in the development of sophisticated motor learning-driven controllers aimed at enhancing gait rehabilitation, we believe that exoskeleton technology remains a sufficiently expansive and fruitful area of research. Given the myriad benefits associated with improved walking ability in patients with CP, as well as the promising functional enhancements reported by various RAGT systems, further exploration in this domain is likely to yield additional advantages for ambulatory function [52]. However, in order to fully clarify the benefits of RAGT, further multicenter studies with large sample sizes and uniform methodologies should be conducted. In addition, further investigation is required to clarify the optimal timing and rehabilitation strategies to maximize gait rehabilitation in patients with CP. Furthermore, we propose that as artificial intelligence progresses, future research should advance toward more structured and standardized investigations to elucidate and expand the RAGT functionalities advantageous for CP patients.

Author details

Lihua Jin[1], Caixia Zhao[2], Binjing Dou[2], Juchuan Dong[1] and Ping He[3*]

1 Department of Rehabilitation Medicine, Second Affiliated Hospital of Kunming Medical University, Kunming, Yunnan, China

2 Department of Pediatrics, Yunnan University of Traditional Chinese Medicine, Kunming, Yunnan, China

3 Department of Pediatrics, First Affiliated Hospital of Yunnan University of Traditional Chinese Medicine, Kunming, Yunnan, China

*Address all correspondence to: hepingx8@sina.com

IntechOpen

References

[1] Vitrikas K, Dalton H, Breish D. Cerebral palsy: An overview. American Family Physician. 2020;**101**(4):213-220

[2] Patel DR et al. Cerebral palsy in children: A clinical overview. Translational pediatrics. 2020;**9** (Suppl. 1):S125

[3] Schless S-H et al. Combining muscle morphology and neuromotor symptoms to explain abnormal gait at the ankle joint level in cerebral palsy. Gait & Posture. 2019;**68**:531-537

[4] Sarajchi M, Al-Hares MK, Sirlantzis K. Wearable lower-limb exoskeleton for children with cerebral palsy: A systematic review of mechanical design, actuation type, control strategy, and clinical evaluation. IEEE Transactions on Neural Systems and Rehabilitation Engineering. 2021;**29**:2695-2720

[5] Wren TA, Rethlefsen S, Kay RM. Prevalence of specific gait abnormalities in children with cerebral palsy: Influence of cerebral palsy subtype, age, and previous surgery. Journal of Pediatric Orthopaedics. 2005;**25**(1):79-83

[6] Kim SW et al. The nature of rehabilitation services provided to children with cerebral palsy: A population-based nationwide study. BMC Health Services Research. 2019;**19**:1-7

[7] Çağlar Okur S, Uğur M, Şenel K. Effects of botulinum toxin a injection on ambulation capacity in patients with cerebral palsy. Developmental Neurorehabilitation. 2019;**22**(4):288-291

[8] Leister KR et al. Neuromuscular contributions to disability in children with cerebral palsy and the impact of dynamic stretching orthoses and therapeutic exercise interventions: A narrative review. Translational Pediatrics. 2024;**13**(5):803

[9] Shin J et al. Comparative effects of passive and active mode robot-assisted gait training on brain and muscular activities in sub-acute and chronic stroke. NeuroRehabilitation. 2022;**51**(1):51-63

[10] Youssofzadeh V et al. Directed functional connectivity in fronto-centroparietal circuit correlates with motor adaptation in gait training. IEEE Transactions on Neural Systems and Rehabilitation Engineering. 2016;**24**(11):1265-1275

[11] Kim DH, Kang CS, Kyeong S. Robot-assisted gait training promotes brain reorganization after stroke: A randomized controlled pilot study. NeuroRehabilitation. 2020;**46**(4):483-489

[12] Kim HY et al. Best facilitated cortical activation during different stepping, treadmill, and robot-assisted walking training paradigms and speeds: A functional near-infrared spectroscopy neuroimaging study. NeuroRehabilitation. 2016;**38**(2):171-178

[13] Tang Z et al. Evidence that robot-assisted gait training modulates neuroplasticity after stroke: An fMRI pilot study based on graph theory analysis. Brain Research. 2024;**1842**:149113

[14] Li Z et al. Adaptive neural control of a kinematically redundant exoskeleton robot using brain–machine interfaces. IEEE Transactions on Neural Networks and Learning Systems. 2018;**30**(12):3558-3571

[15] Colombo G et al. Treadmill training of paraplegic patients using a robotic orthosis. Journal of Rehabilitation Research and Development. 2000;**37**(6):693-700

[16] Carvalho I et al. Robotic gait training for individuals with cerebral palsy: A systematic review and meta-analysis. Archives of Physical Medicine and Rehabilitation. 2017;**98**(11):2332-2344

[17] Lefmann S, Russo R, Hillier S. The effectiveness of robotic-assisted gait training for paediatric gait disorders: Systematic review. Journal of Neuroengineering and Rehabilitation. 2017;**14**:1-10

[18] Hidler JM, Wall AE. Alterations in muscle activation patterns during robotic-assisted walking. Clinical biomechanics. 2005;**20**(2):184-193

[19] Bayon C et al. Development and evaluation of a novel robotic platform for gait rehabilitation in patients with cerebral palsy: CPWalker. Robotics and Autonomous Systems. 2017;**91**:101-114

[20] Bayón C et al. Locomotor training through a novel robotic platform for gait rehabilitation in pediatric population. Journal of Neuroengineering and Rehabilitation. 2016;**13**:1-6

[21] Grodon C, Bassett P, Shannon H. The 'heROIC' trial: Does the use of a robotic rehabilitation trainer change quality of life, range of movement and function in children with cerebral palsy? Child: Care Health and Development. 2023;**49**(5):914-924

[22] Choi JY et al. Training intensity of robot-assisted gait training in children with cerebral palsy. Developmental Medicine & Child Neurology. 2024;**66**(8):1096-1105

[23] Kitatani R et al. Reduction in energy expenditure during walking using an automated stride assistance device in healthy young adults. Archives of Physical Medicine and Rehabilitation. 2014;**95**(11):2128-2133

[24] Wessels M et al. Body weight-supported gait training for restoration of walking in people with an incomplete spinal cord injury: A systematic review. Journal of Rehabilitation Medicine. 2010;**42**(6):513-519

[25] Conner BC, Remec NM, Lerner ZF. Is robotic gait training effective for individuals with cerebral palsy? A systematic review and meta-analysis of randomized controlled trials. Clinical Rehabilitation. 2022;**36**(7):873-882

[26] Borggraefe I et al. Robotic-assisted treadmill therapy improves walking and standing performance in children and adolescents with cerebral palsy. European Journal of Paediatric Neurology. 2010;**14**(6):496-502

[27] Algabbani MF et al. Effect of robotic-assisted gait training program on spatiotemporal gait parameters for ambulatory children with cerebral palsy: A randomized control trial. NeuroRehabilitation. 2024;**55**(1):127-136

[28] Willoughby KL et al. Efficacy of partial body weight–supported treadmill training compared with overground walking practice for children with cerebral palsy: A randomized controlled trial. Archives of Physical Medicine and Rehabilitation. 2010;**91**(3):333-339

[29] Jin P, Wang Y. The impact of botulinum toxin combined with robotassisted gait training on spasticity and gross motor function on children with spastic cerebral palsy. Developmental Neurorehabilitation. 2024;**27**(5-6):155-160

[30] Fu W-S et al. Virtual reality combined with robot-assisted gait training to improve walking ability of children with cerebral palsy: A randomized controlled trial. Technology and Health Care. 2022;**30**(6):1525-1533

[31] Kawamura K et al. Effect of a weekly functional independence measure scale on the recovery of patient with acute stroke: A retrospective study. Medicine. 2022;**101**(11):e28974

[32] Mak M. Repetitive transcranial magnetic stimulation combined with treadmill training can modulate corticomotor inhibition and improve walking performance in people with Parkinson's disease. Journal of Physiotherapy. 2013;**59**(2):128-128

[33] Duarte NDAC et al. Effect of transcranial direct-current stimulation combined with treadmill training on balance and functional performance in children with cerebral palsy: A double-blind randomized controlled trial. PLoS One. 2014;**9**(8):e105777

[34] Delgado E et al. ATLAS2030 pediatric gait exoskeleton: Changes on range of motion, strength and spasticity in children with cerebral palsy. A case series study. Frontiers in Pediatrics. 2021;**9**:753226

[35] Schmidt-Lucke C et al. Effect of assisted walking-movement in patients with genetic and acquired neuromuscular disorders with the motorised Innowalk device: An international case study meta-analysis. PeerJ. 2019;**7**:e7098

[36] Lerner ZF et al. A robotic exoskeleton for treatment of crouch gait in children with cerebral palsy: Design and initial application. IEEE Transactions on Neural Systems and Rehabilitation Engineering. 2016;**25**(6):650-659

[37] Kuroda MM et al. Benefits of a wearable cyborg HAL (hybrid assistive limb) in patients with childhood-onset motor disabilities: A 1-year follow-up study. Pediatric Reports. 2023;**15**(1):215-226

[38] Chen J et al. A pediatric knee exoskeleton with real-time adaptive control for overground walking in ambulatory individuals with cerebral palsy. Frontiers in Robotics and AI. 2021;**8**:702137

[39] Aboutorabi A et al. Efficacy of ankle foot orthoses types on walking in children with cerebral palsy: A systematic review. Annals of Physical and Rehabilitation Medicine. 2017;**60**(6):393-402

[40] Lerner ZF et al. An untethered ankle exoskeleton improves walking economy in a pilot study of individuals with cerebral palsy. IEEE Transactions on Neural Systems and Rehabilitation Engineering. 2018;**26**(10):1985-1993

[41] Roth EJ et al. Hemiplegic gait: Relationships between walking speed and other temporal parameters: 1. American Journal of Physical Medicine & Rehabilitation. 1997;**76**(2): 128-133

[42] Lee J et al. Effects of a lower limb rehabilitation robot with various training modes in patients with stroke: A randomized controlled trial. Medicine. 2022;**101**(44):e31590

[43] Marchal-Crespo L, Riener R. Robot-assisted gait training. In: Rehabilitation Robotics. Academic Press, Elsevier; 2018. pp. 227-240

[44] Wang X et al. A multistage hemiplegic lower-limb rehabilitation robot: Design and gait trajectory planning. Sensors. 2024;**24**(7):2310

[45] Hu C et al. Effect of acupuncture combined with lower limb gait rehabilitation robot on improving walking function in stroke patients with hemiplegia. Neuro Rehabilitation. 2024;**54**(2):309-317

[46] DeVol CR et al. Effects of spinal stimulation and short-burst treadmill training on gait biomechanics in children with cerebral palsy. Gait & Posture. 2025;**118**:25-32

[47] Shepherd et al. Evaluating the use of electromyography in UK and European gait laboratories for the assessment of cerebral palsy and other neurological and musculoskeletal conditions. Gait & Posture. 2025;**117**:143-152

[48] Zhou Z et al. Mechatronic design of an ankle-foot rehabilitation robot for children with cerebral palsy and preliminary clinical trial. Toronto, ON, Canada: 2017 IEEE International Conference on Industrial Technology (ICIT); 2017. pp. 825-830

[49] Wang R et al. A preliminary clinical study on robot-assisted ankle rehabilitation of children with cerebral palsy. Journal of Peking University (Medical Science). 2018;**50**(2):207-212

[50] Chung BPH. Effectiveness of robotic-assisted gait training in stroke rehabilitation: A retrospective matched control study. Hong Kong Physiotherapy Journal. 2017;**36**:10-16

[51] Mazzucchelli M et al. Evidence-based improvement of gait in post-stroke patients following robot-assisted training: A systematic review. NeuroRehabilitation. 2022;**51**(4):595-608

[52] Marks D et al. The Andago for overground gait training in patients with gait disorders after stroke-results from a usability study. Physiotherapy Research and Reports. 2019;**2**(2):1-8

Chapter 5

Hand Splinting

N.S. Krishna and S.G. Praveen

Abstract

Cerebral palsy often results in impaired hand function, limiting an individual's ability to participate in daily activities and impacting their overall quality of life. Hand splinting is a crucial therapeutic intervention that can significantly enhance hand function, reduce deformity, and promote independence. However, effective hand splinting requires a comprehensive understanding of the underlying principles, techniques, and considerations. This chapter provides a detailed and practical guide to hand splinting for individuals with cerebral palsy. It covers the various types of hand splints, including their indications, advantages, and limitations. The chapter also discusses essential considerations and tips in splint making, assessment, and fitting to ensure optimal outcomes. Additionally, it outlines wearing schedules and strategies for promoting compliance and effective use. Finally, the chapter highlights recent advancements in hand splinting, providing readers with a comprehensive understanding of current best practices. By combining theory, practical guidance, and evidence-based recommendations, this chapter serves as an invaluable resource for healthcare professionals seeking to enhance hand function and improve the lives of individuals with cerebral palsy. The information presented in this chapter will enable occupational therapists, physiotherapists, and other healthcare professionals to design and implement effective hand splinting interventions, ultimately improving the functional abilities and quality of life of individuals with cerebral palsy.

Keywords: cerebral palsy, hand splinting, splint, orthotics, neurological recovery, rehabilitation, hand function

1. Introduction

Hand splinting is a pivotal intervention in managing children with cerebral palsy (CP), a condition marked by motor impairments resulting from non-progressive disturbances in the developing brain. The upper limbs, particularly the hands, are often significantly affected, leading to challenges in achieving functional independence. Abnormal postures, such as thumb adduction and wrist flexion, can impede the ability to perform daily activities, necessitating effective management strategies [1].

The primary objective of hand splinting is to enhance hand function by addressing muscle tone irregularities, joint alignment issues, and overall dexterity. Splints serve a variety of purposes, including immobilizing joints to prevent contractures, providing support during functional tasks, and facilitating movement through dynamic designs. Consequently, they are not only instrumental in improving physical capabilities but also in promoting meaningful participation in daily activities.

Recent reviews suggest that while hand splints can yield moderate improvements in upper limb skills when combined with therapy, these benefits often diminish once splint use is discontinued [2]. This highlights the importance of integrating splinting within a comprehensive therapeutic framework tailored to each child's specific needs. Additionally, the implementation of splinting requires careful consideration of potential drawbacks, such as discomfort and esthetic concerns.

This chapter delves into the principles of hand splinting for children with CP, focusing on splint types, fabrication techniques, and evidence-based practices. Furthermore, it explores emerging trends in splint design, including advancements in 3D printing technology. By gaining a nuanced understanding of hand splinting, occupational therapists can better support children with cerebral palsy in achieving their functional goals and enhancing their quality of life.

2. Understanding splint: Definition and its application

Mosby's Medical, Nursing, and Allied Health Dictionary (2002) defines a splint as "an orthopedic device for immobilization, restraint, or support of any body part" [3].

The text also defines orthosis as "a force system designed to control, correct, or compensate for a bone deformity, deforming forces, or forces absent from the body" [4] Today, these healthcare field terms are often used synonymously. Technically, the term splint refers to a temporary device that is part of a treatment program. In contrast, the term orthosis refers to a permanent device to replace or substitute for loss of muscle function.

Splints and orthoses not only immobilize but also mobilize, position, and protect a joint or specific body part. Splints range in design and fabrication from simple to complex, depending on the goals established for a particular condition [5].

In CP, hand splints may be commonly used as a therapeutic modality to assist with developmentally meaningful skills. Hand splints (orthoses or upper limb splints) are removable external devices designed to support a weak or ineffective joint or muscle. Under the ICF framework, hand splints may be classified as an environmental factor (such as physical support) influencing the overall interaction of ICF domains that can impact a child's body function and structure as well as activity and participation [4].

3. Aims of hand splinting

- Prevent contractures and joint deformities.

- Maintain joint integrity and ROM.

- Balance muscle tone and reduce hypertonicity.

- Position limbs for functional use.

- Manage pain, edema, and hygiene.

- Enhance cosmesis and appearance [5].

4. Assessment and goal setting

Before implementing splinting interventions, a comprehensive assessment must be conducted [6]. This includes evaluating:

- Range of motion

- Muscle tone

- Functional abilities

- Specific goals related to daily activities

The use of a Standardized Scale like MACS (Manual Ability Classification System) is recommended for a comprehensive assessment [7].

4.1 Levels of manual ability classification system (MACS) scale

Handles objects easily and successfully. At most, limitations in the ease of performing manual tasks require speed and accuracy. However, any limitations in manual abilities do not restrict independence in daily activities [7].

Handles most objects but with somewhat reduced quality and/or speed of achievement. Certain activities may be avoided or be achieved with some difficulty, alternative ways of performance might be used but manual abilities do not usually restrict independence in daily activities.

Handles objects with difficulty and needs help to prepare and/or modify activities. The performance is slow and achieved with limited success regarding quality and quantity. Activities are performed independently if they have been set up or adapted.

Handles a limited selection of easily managed objects in adapted situations. Performs parts of activities with effort and with limited success. Requires continuous support and assistance and/or adapted equipment, for even partial achievement of the activity.

Does not handle objects and has severely limited ability to perform even simple actions. Requires total assistance.

The *goal-setting process* for hand splinting involves identifying the individual's specific hand function deficits and priorities, and then setting Specific, Measurable, Achievable, Relevant, and Time-bound (SMART) goals [8] focused on improving hand positioning, range of motion, strength, dexterity, and functional ability. Goals may target specific hand splinting outcomes, such as reducing contractures, improving grasp and release, or enhancing finger isolation, and are regularly reviewed and revised every 3-6 months to assess progress, identify challenges, and adjust the splinting intervention as needed [8].

Setting clear, measurable (SMART) goals is essential for evaluating the effectiveness of the splinting intervention.

5. Considerations for splint design

1. The desired joint position should be clearly defined before starting the splint fabrication process to ensure the splint will support proper alignment and effectively address the needs of children with cerebral palsy [3].

2. The splint should be designed to counteract deforming forces and maintain proper joint alignment, which is crucial for managing deformities in children with cerebral palsy [4].

3. Liners should be used to reduce friction and protect the skin from irritation, particularly when the splint is worn for extended periods [4].

4. A NuStim wrap provides additional cushioning, enhancing patient comfort and supporting skin protection during prolonged splint use [3].

5. Applying a powder like Curash helps control moisture and prevent skin breakdown, which is essential for children with sensitive skin [3].

6. Each joint should be molded individually for better accuracy and fit, reheating and remolding the material as necessary to achieve the desired position and support.

7. Strapping should be adjusted to keep the limb securely within the splint, especially when aiming to reduce hypertonicity or manage contractures.

8. Proper strapping prevents the splint from slipping distally, ensuring it remains in the correct position and maintains its therapeutic effectiveness [4].

9. The strapping system should allow free movement of unaffected joints to enhance functionality and reduce unnecessary restrictions.

10. Straps should be placed carefully to avoid excessive pressure on bony prominences, which could lead to discomfort or skin damage.

11. Wider straps help distribute pressure more evenly, improving comfort and reducing the risk of pressure sores, particularly for children with cerebral palsy [3].

12. Care should be taken to avoid hyperextension in vulnerable joints like the thumb MCP, PIP joints, and the first web space, which are prone to deformities in children with cerebral palsy [3].

13. The design should focus on preserving the first web space and the natural arches of the hand to support proper hand function, which is crucial for children with cerebral palsy.

14. Finger dividers made from materials like thermoplastic, sponge, or Otoform K should be used to create comfortable, functional dividers that prevent contractures and promote hand function [4].

15. A splint with an extended lever arm requires less force to achieve the desired therapeutic effect, making it easier to manage muscle tone and deformities in children with cerebral palsy.

16. Adding contours to the splint design enhances strength and durability, reducing bulk while improving comfort and support.

17. Distributing pressure over a larger surface area decreases discomfort and reduces the risk of skin breakdown, which is particularly important for children with cerebral palsy.

18. The splint design should balance opposing forces to provide stability and functional positioning, helping improve mobility and prevent deformities in children with cerebral palsy [3].

Thus, splints for children with cerebral palsy should ensure proper joint alignment, comfort, and functionality, with features such as customized molding, secure strapping, and skin protection. Design elements such as pressure distribution, preserved hand arches, and balanced forces enhance therapeutic effectiveness and prevent deformities.

6. Hints for orthotic fabrication for children with increased tone

Fabricating an orthosis on a child with increased tone is challenging with experience, therapists gain insight into methods that optimize the process. The following are hints [4] for the novice therapist who is fabricating an orthosis for a child with increased tone:

- Choose a quiet location, and minimize other activities.

- Be conscious of lighting and room temperature.

- Invite parents/caregivers to assist if they can calmly help.

- Position the child comfortably so that muscle tone is as close to normal as possible.

- Speak calmly and slowly, and handle the child's extremity gently

- Use soft music, sing, or read a story for a calming effect.

- Do not use toys to distract the child because they can cause overexcitement, resulting tone a crossover effect and increase.

- Prevent any sudden quick movements.

- Have parents assist in keeping the arm and specifically the elbow stable on the surface.

- Avoid touching the palm. First, abduct the thumb out of the palm, and flex the wrist to normalize tone as much as possible. Then try extending the wrist while avoiding the palm as much as possible.

7. Splint-wearing schedule for hypertonicity

The splint-wearing schedule for individuals with hypertonicity, especially children with cerebral palsy, should be tailored to manage muscle tone effectively and promote functional balance [7]. Below are the recommended schedules for different levels of hypertonicity (Refer **Table 1**):

Condition	Schedule
Continuous low-load stretch	Apply a gentle, consistent stretch through splints to reduce spasticity and muscle tone, ideally for extended periods during the day or night.
Encourage antagonist muscle use	Regularly remove the splint to allow active use of antagonist muscles, promoting functional balance and muscle control.
Contractures	Combine night splinting with daytime use or other interventions to optimize results in managing hypertonicity and preventing muscle contractures.
Mild hypertonicity	Use splints during short activity sessions for individuals whose hypertonicity appears only during activity, enhancing control and preventing excessive muscle tightness.
Severe hypertonicity	Prolonged splint use is recommended for individuals with moderate-to-severe hypertonicity even at rest to maintain joint alignment and reduce tone.

Table 1.
Hand splinting schedules for different levels of hypertonicity.

This schedule ensures a balanced approach to managing hypertonicity, allowing for proper muscle function and effective reduction of spasticity.

8. Categories of hand splints

In the management of children with cerebral palsy (CP), a wide range of hand splints constructed from various materials are employed in clinical practice. These splints generally serve two overarching purposes, aligning with distinct domains of the International Classification of Functioning, Disability, and Health (ICF): the *body function and structure domain* and the *activity and participation domain* (**Figure 1**) [4].

8.1 Non-functional hand splints

The first category, *non-functional hand splints* [3], primarily focuses on improving outcomes related to the body function and structure domain of the ICF. These splints are designed to address issues such as muscle contractures, abnormal muscle tone, and joint deformities.
Examples include:

- *Resting hand splints*: These are used to prevent or correct muscle contractures by maintaining the hand in a neutral or stretched position.

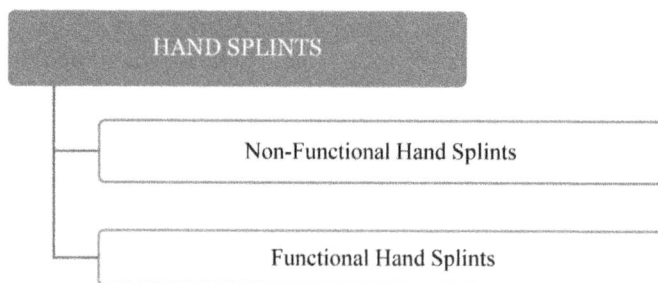

Figure 1.
Categories of hand splints.

- *Supination casts*: These are employed to lengthen muscles or inhibit excessive muscle tone [4].

Due to their design, non-functional splints often restrict voluntary hand movements, making them unsuitable for use during daily activities. As a result, they are typically worn at night or for short durations (i.e., for a week) to achieve specific therapeutic goals, such as increasing muscle length or reducing muscle tightness.

Non-functional splints can also be categorized based on their intended duration of use:

- *Removable splints*: Prescribed for long-term use, these splints aim to stretch muscles over time, serving as a preventive measure against contractures.

- *Serial casts*: These are applied for short-term use to achieve immediate muscle stretching while minimizing potential adverse effects, such as muscle weakness due to prolonged immobilization. The expectation is that serial casting will result in medium- to long-term improvements in muscle length following the removal of the cast [4].

8.2 Functional hand splints

The second category, *functional hand splints* [3], is designed to enhance the outcomes in the activity and participation domain of the ICF. These splints support specific functional tasks and activities by improving upper limb positioning and stability, enabling children to better perform activities such as writing, feeding, or other daily tasks. An example of a functional splint is the *Wrist Cock-Up Splint*, which stabilizes the wrist joint and positions it optimally during functional activities, such as handwriting or utensil use during meals.

Unlike non-functional splints, functional splints are worn during task performance to promote engagement in meaningful activities. They are prescribed to facilitate optimal functional outcomes by improving the biomechanics of upper limb movements.

9. Hand splints widely used for cerebral palsy

9.1 Functional resting splint

- This splint is commonly recommended for individuals with moderate-to-severe increased tone or significantly decreased tone.

- It prevents contractures and maintains hygiene by positioning the wrist at 30° extension, metacarpophalangeal joints at 50° flexion, and interphalangeal joints at a progressive 10°-30° flexion (**Figure 2**) [4].

9.2 Wrist extension splint

- It is used to support wrist extension in individuals with cerebral palsy, this splint is designed to maintain alignment.

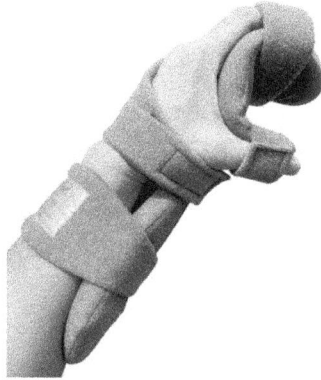

Figure 2.
Functional resting splint.

- Research indicates that neutral wrist splints are generally more acceptable to patients, with higher compliance levels compared to wrist extension splints (**Figure 3**) [4].

9.3 Weight-bearing splint

- This splint aids in therapeutic activities requiring weight-bearing.

- It positions the wrist in approximately 90° extension and aligns the digits for stability.

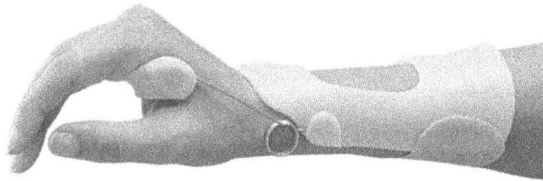

Figure 3.
Wrist extension splint.

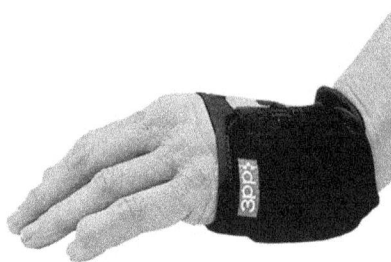

Figure 4.
Weight-bearing splint.

- It is particularly valuable during therapy sessions focused on improving weight-bearing tasks (**Figure 4**) [6].

9.4 Anti-spasticity splint

- Highly effective in addressing spasticity, this splint facilitates wrist extension, finger abduction, and thumb abduction using finger troughs.

- Its benefits include positioning the hand functionally, improving hygiene, and applying prolonged stretch (**Figure 5**) [6].

9.5 Serpentine splint

Designed to minimize thumb adduction contractures, this splint wraps around the thumb from the hypothenar region, across the dorsum, and through the web space to the thenar eminence.

- It allows wrist movement while providing thumb stability during functional activities, effectively preventing deformities (**Figure 6**) [4].

9.6 Volar splint

- The resting volar splint was one of the earliest splint designs that attempted to reduce spasticity by placing a muscle under constant stretch with increased tone.

- Targets muscle spindles to reduce their sensitivity to stretching, potentially improving motor control in individuals with cerebral palsy (CP).

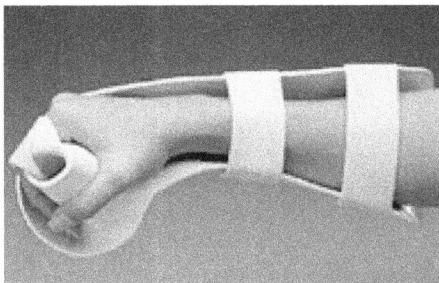

Figure 5.
Anti-spasticity splint.

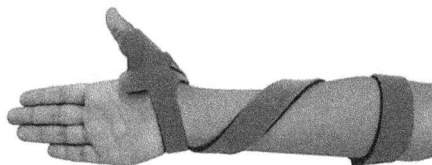

Figure 6.
Serpentine splint.

- Commonly used for managing wrist and finger flexor spasticity in CP [4].

9.7 Dorsal splint

- Facilitates extensor muscle activation by stimulating the dorsal forearm while inhibiting flexor muscles.

- Particularly beneficial in CP cases with excessive wrist and finger flexion due to spasticity.

- Enhances balance between flexors and extensors for improved hand positioning (**Figure 7**) [4].

9.8 Finger spreader

- A foam device is recommended to encourage finger extension and inhibit flexor spasticity.

- Prevents the hand from assuming a tight fist posture, a common issue in children with CP.

- Supports better functional hand positioning for daily tasks (**Figure 8**) [4].

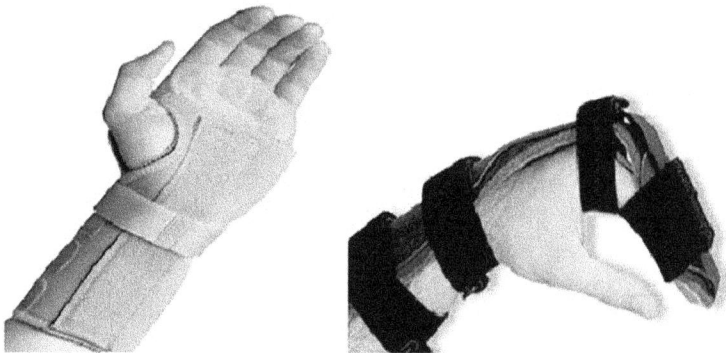

Figure 7.
Volar and dorsal splint.

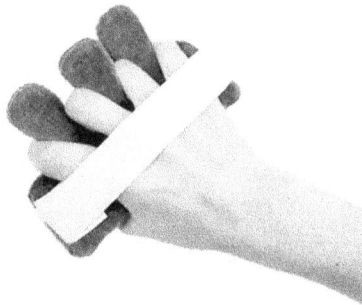

Figure 8.
Finger spreader.

9.9 Firm cone

- Inserted in the palm to counteract flexor spasticity by applying pressure to the flexor surfaces.

- Useful for managing severe hand spasticity in CP but requires careful monitoring to avoid excessive pressure or discomfort.

- Helps open the hand, enabling better hygiene and functional engagement (**Figure 9**) [6].

9.10 MacKinnon splint

- Applies pressure on the volar side of the metacarpal heads, activating intrinsic hand muscles.

- Reduces tone in the adductor pollicis and finger flexors, improving thumb and finger positioning in CP.

- Supports functional hand use by facilitating grasp and release actions (**Figure 10**) [6].

9.11 Orthokinetic cuff

- The system was created using an Ace bandage with both elastic and nonelastic components.

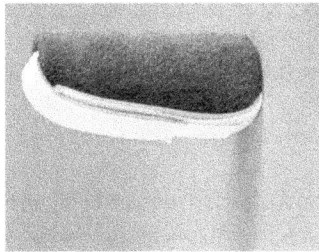

Figure 9.
Firm cone splint.

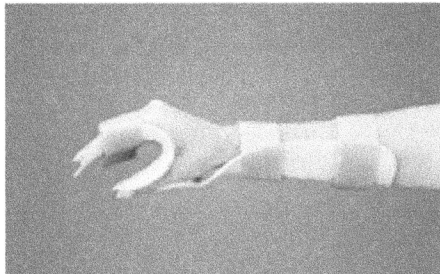

Figure 10.
MacKinnon splint.

- It was constructed using a variation of the continuous fold-over method, consisting of three layers.

- Nonelastic Velfoam was sewn into the pieces, and the cuff was designed to fit snugly around the upper forearm, aligning with the muscle bellies of the wrist and finger extensors in the elastic (active) area [4].

- It helps reduce spasticity and improve voluntary movement in children with cerebral palsy (CP). The design enhances wrist extension, facilitating functional activities such as reaching and grasping [6].

9.12 Short opponens thumb splint

- This splint was made of arthroplasty, with particular consideration provided to holding the thumb out of palmar adduction-opposition by having leverage over the eminence of the thenar.

- Both the thumb MP and IP joints were strengthened but enough of the thumb pad was left exposed to allow an opposite grip to be used.

- The orthoplast proceeded over the hand dorsum, stopping over the eminence of the hypothenar. This portion has been stabilized with a Velcro strap to the thumb portion (**Figure 11**) [4].

9.13 Lycra orthoses

- In the last 10 years, many types of Lycra-based orthosis have emerged, with styles ranging from full-body suits to smaller garments such as sleeves/gloves and leggings. Children with CP demonstrate practical benefits when using Lycra orthosis as they provide compression and proprioceptive feedback.

- Improve postural control and upper limb function in children with CP.

- The versatile design supports both gross and fine motor tasks by enhancing muscle alignment and reducing involuntary movements [4].

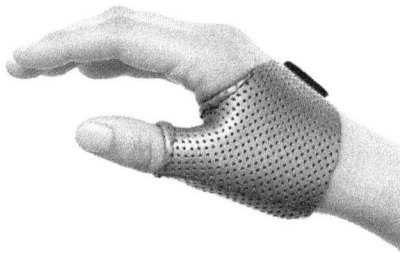

Figure 11.
Short opponens thumb splint.

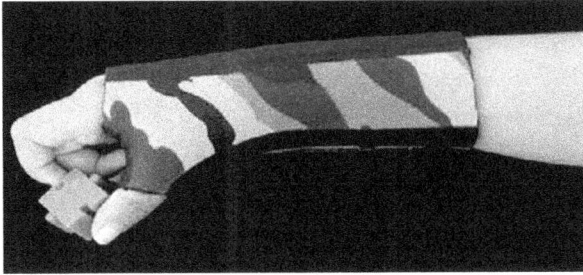

Figure 12.
WETA orthosis.

9.14 WETA orthosis (wrist extension thumb abduction orthosis)

- Specifically designed to counteract spastic patterns such as wrist flexion, ulnar deviation, and thumb adduction in CP (i.e., a hand that experiences wrist flexion, ulnar deviation, ulnar flexion, and thumb adduction).

- Enhances hand positioning for improved grasp and manipulation of objects.

- Effective in promoting wrist stability and facilitating purposeful hand use in hypertonic conditions (**Figure 12**) [6].

10. Innovations in design

Recent advancements have introduced concepts such as *tone-reducing, inhibitive, neurophysiological, or dynamic designs* for casts, splints, and orthoses. These designs aim to influence spasticity and muscle tone, offering potential therapeutic benefits. While widely adopted in certain clinical settings, there is currently insufficient evidence to confirm their superiority over traditional biomechanical designs.

10.1 Recent advances in hand splinting

3D-printed dynamic upper extremity orthoses (DUEOs) are transforming the management of children with cerebral palsy by providing highly customized solutions that enhance both comfort and functionality [9]. For example: A 3D-printed finger splint was made to correct the dystonia-induced swan neck and Boutonniere deformities.

Unlike traditional orthotic devices, which can be cumbersome and less adaptable, 3D-printed orthoses are lightweight and specifically tailored to fit the unique anatomy of each child. This level of personalization not only improves the overall fit but also optimizes pressure distribution, thereby reducing the risk of skin irritation and enhancing user compliance [9].

In addition to their comfort advantages, 3D-printed orthoses demonstrate notable durability and ease of modification. The advanced materials utilized in 3D printing are engineered to withstand regular use while maintaining structural integrity over time. Moreover, the rapid production capabilities inherent in 3D printing allow for swift adjustments to the orthosis as a child's needs evolve, ensuring ongoing effectiveness throughout their development. Overall, 3D-printed dynamic upper extremity orthoses represent a significant advancement in orthotic technology, integrating enhanced comfort with functional support to improve the quality of life for children with upper extremity impairments.

11. Hand-based adaptations in cerebral palsy

Individuals with cerebral palsy often experience hand function deficits, impacting their ability to participate in daily activities. Hand-based adaptations, including splinting and assistive technology, play a crucial role in enhancing hand function, independence, and quality of life.

11.1 HAAT model

The Human Activity Assistive Technology (HAAT) model provides a framework for understanding the complex interactions between the individual, activity, and assistive technology. This model guides the selection and implementation of hand-based adaptations, ensuring a person-centered approach [10].

11.2 Hand-based adaptations

In addition to splinting, various hand-based adaptations can be used to enhance hand function and independence:

1. Adaptive utensils and devices [10]: Utensils with angled or bent handles, contoured or thickened handles, or lightweight materials.

2. Assistive technology [10]: Adaptive keyboards, mouse devices, and tablet or smartphone adaptations.

3. Daily living aids [10]: Dressing aids, bathing aids, and feeding aids with adapted handles or grips.

4. Recreational and leisure aids [10]: Adaptive sports equipment, hobby aids, and game and puzzle aids.

11.3 Intervention implementation

Effective implementation and monitoring of hand-based adaptations requires a comprehensive individualized assessment to identify strengths, needs, and goals. A device trial and evaluation ensure proper fit and effectiveness. Training and education on device use and maintenance are provided to the individual, family, and caregivers. Regular follow-up and monitoring enable adjustments and ensure continued effectiveness, ultimately enhancing hand function, independence, and quality of life for individuals with cerebral palsy.

12. Chapter summary

This chapter provides a comprehensive guide to hand splinting for individuals with cerebral palsy. It discusses the need for splinting in individuals with CP. The chapter covers various aspects of hand splinting, including types of splints, considerations, and tips for splint making, assessment, goal setting, and wearing schedules. Additionally, it highlights recent advancements in hand splinting, aiming to equip healthcare professionals with the knowledge and skills necessary to improve hand function and quality of life for individuals with cerebral palsy.

Acronyms and abbreviations

CP	Cerebral Palsy
ICF	International Classification of Functioning, Disability, and Health
MACS	Manual Ability Classification System
SMART	Specific, Measurable, Achievable, Relevant, and Time-bound
DUEOs	Dynamic Upper Extremity Orthoses

Author details

N.S. Krishna* and S.G. Praveen
KMCH College of Occupational Therapy, Coimbatore, India

*Address all correspondence to: drkrishnansk@gmail.com;
krishna.ns@kmchcot.ac.in

IntechOpen

References

[1] The upper limb in cerebral palsy. Hand Clinics. 2003;**19**:4

[2] Basu AP, Pearse J, Kelly S, Wisher V, Kisler J. Early intervention to improve hand function in hemiplegic cerebral palsy. Frontiers in Neurology. 2015;**5**:281. DOI: 10.3389/fneur.2014.00281IF:2.7Q2B3

[3] Coppard B, Lohman H. Introduction to Splinting: A Clinical Reasoning and Problem-Solving Approach. 3rd ed. St. Louis: Mosby Elsevier; 2008

[4] Coppard BM, Lohman H. Introduction to Orthotics: A Clinical Reasoning and Problem-Solving Approach. 5th ed. St. Louis: Mosby Elsevier; 2019

[5] Jackman M, Novak I, Lannin N. Effectiveness of hand splints in children with cerebral palsy: A systematic review with meta-analysis. Developmental Medicine and Child Neurology. 2014;**56**(2):138-147. DOI: 10.1111/dmcn.12205

[6] Case-Smith J, O'Brien JC. Occupational Therapy for Children and Adolescents. 8th ed. St. Louis: Elsevier; 2020

[7] Eliasson et al. The manual ability classification system (MACS) for children with cerebral palsy: Scale development and evidence of validity and reliability. Developmental Medicine and Child Neurology. 2006;**48**:549-554

[8] Crepeau EB, Cohn ES, Schell BAB. Willard and Spackman's Occupational Therapy. 10th ed. Philadelphia: Lippincott Williams & Wilkins; 2003

[9] Yang YS, Tseng CH, Fang WC, Han IW, Huang SC. Effectiveness of a new 3D-printed dynamic hand-wrist splint on hand motor function and spasticity in chronic stroke patients. Journal of Clinical Medicine. 2021;**10**(19):4549. DOI: 10.3390/jcm10194549

[10] Christiansen CH, Baum CM, Bass JD. Occupational Therapy: Performance, Participation, and Well-Being. 4th ed. SLACK Incorporated: Thorofare (NJ); 2015